ROLE OF MEDROXYPROGESTERONE IN ENDOCRINE-RELATED TUMORS

VOLUME 2

Role of Medroxyprogesterone in Endocrine-Related Tumors

Volume 2

Editors

L. Campio, M.D.
Division of Medical Affairs
The Upjohn Company
Kalamazoo, Michigan

G. Robustelli Della Cuna, M.D.
Head of the Divison of Oncology
Clinica del Lavoro Foundation
University of Pavia
Pavia, Italy

R. W. Taylor, M.D., F.R.C.O.G.
Head of the Department of Gynaecology
St. Thomas's Hospital Medical School
University of London
London, United Kingdom

Raven Press ■ New York

Raven Press, 1140 Avenue of the Americas, New York, New York 10036

Made in the United States of America

Library of Congress Cataloging in Publication Data
Main entry under title:

Role of medroxyprogesterone in endocrine-related tumors.

    "Volume 2."
    Includes bibliographical references and index.
    1. Medroxyprogesterone—Testing—Congresses.
2. Cancer—Chemotherapy—Congresses. 3. Breast—
Cancer—Chemotherapy—Congresses. I. Campio, L.
II. Robustelli Della Cuna, Gioacchino. III. Taylor, R. W.
(Ronald Wentworth) [DNLM: 1. Breast neoplasms—Drug
therapy—Congresses. 2. Uterine neoplasms—Drug therapy
—Congresses. 3. Medroxyprogesterone—Therapeutics—
Congresses. 4. Medroxyprogesterone—Pharmacodynamics—
Congresses. WP   530 R745   1981]
RC271.M35R64   1983   616.99′4449061   82-40295
ISBN 0-89004-865-7

    Great care has been taken to maintain the accuracy of the information contained in the volume. However, Raven Press cannot be held responsible for errors or for any consequences arising from the use of the information contained herein.

Preface

Renewed interest in hormonal therapy of endocrine-related tumors has resulted from new information about estrogen and progesterone receptors and host–tumor endocrine correlations, as well as the availability of new drugs.

Based on the assumption that tumors of endocrine-sensitive tissues may retain the hormone sensitivity of the original cell type, a number of endocrine manipulations have been used in the management of breast, endometrial, and prostatic cancer. The discovery of hormone receptors in ovarian carcinoma suggests that this tumor might also respond to treatment with hormone therapy.

This volume focuses on the use of one such hormone, medroxyprogesterone acetate, whose importance in the treatment of several hormone-sensitive tumors has resulted from its multiple modes of action on the tumor. Chapters discuss pharmacokinetics of the drug, its effects on tumor cell proliferation, the rationale for combined antiestrogen plus progestin therapy, comparisons of effects with different dosage levels and combinations, and specific studies with tumors of several estrogen sensitive tumor types.

The volume will be of interest to medical oncologists, endocrinologists and urologists who manage endocrine-sensitive tumors, and to biologists and pharmacologists involved in the development of new antitumor agents and the study of basic tumor cell function.

The Editors

Acknowledgments

The meeting on which this book is based has been organized with the financial contribution of The Upjohn Company. Our thanks also go to everybody who cooperated with the organization of the meeting and with the publication of the book, in particular to M. G. R.-Milan for the organization of the symposium and to Mrs. P. Simoni and Miss M. Comotti for their help in the preparation of the manuscripts.

Contents

1   Inhibitory Effects of Medroxyprogesterone Acetate on the
     Proliferation of Human Breast Cancer Cells
     S. Iacobelli, G. Sica, C. Natoli, and D. Gatti

7   DNA Flow Cytometry of the Endometrium
     Arnold C. M. van Lindert, George P. J. Alsbach, and
     Derk H. Rutgers

15 A Rationale for Combined Antiestrogen plus Progestin
     Administration in Breast Cancer
     Etienne-Emile Baulieu

19 Pharmacokinetics of Oral Medroxyprogesterone Acetate at
     Moderate Doses in a Long-Term Study
     P. Periti, M. Ciuffi, and T. Mazzei

25 Pharmacokinetics of Medroxyprogesterone Acetate and Plasma
     Levels in a Long-Term Treatment
     Inge Hesselius

35 High-Dose Medroxyprogesterone Acetate Therapy: Plasma Levels
     and Bioavailability-Response Correlation After Single and
     Multiple Dose Administration in Advanced Cancer Patients—
     Preliminary Results
     F. Pannuti, C. M. Camaggi, E. Strocchi, M. Giovannini,
     G. Iafelice, A. Lippi, N. Canova, and B. Costanti

45 Medroxyprogesterone Acetate and Tamoxifen: Two Different Drugs
     in Alternate or Sequential Modality Treatment
     A. Pellegrini, B. Massidda, V. Mascia, and M. T. Ionta

69 Low- Versus High-Dose Medroxyprogesterone Acetate in the
     Treatment of Advanced Breast Cancer
     F. Cavalli, A. Goldhirsch, F. Jungi, G. Martz, and P. Alberto

77 Medroxyprogesterone Acetate at Two Different High Doses for the
     Treatment of Advanced Breast Cancer
     H. Cortés Funes, P. L. Madrigal, G. Perez Mangas, and
     C. Mendiola

85 High-Dose Medroxyprogesterone Acetate in Metastatic Breast
   Cancer: Preliminary Report on Three AIO Phase II Trials
   H.-E. Wander, H.-H. Bartsch, H.-Ch. Blossey, and G.A. Nagel

95 The Results of Treatment with Medroxyprogesterone Acetate at
   High and Very High Doses in 237 Metastatic Breast Cancer
   Patients in Postmenopause
   F. Pannuti, M.R.A. Gentili, A.R. Di Marco, A. Martoni,
   M.E. Giambiasi, R. Battistoni, C.M. Camaggi, P. Burroni,
   E. Strocchi, G. Iafelice, E. Piana, and G. Murari

105 Oral or Intramuscular Treatment of Advanced Breast Cancer with
    Medroxyprogesterone Acetate: A Review
    J. Løber, H.T. Mouridsen, and C. Rose

115 Medroxyprogesterone Acetate High Dose and Bromocriptine:
    Results of a 4-Year Study in Stage IV Breast Cancer
    L. Dogliotti, A. Mussa, and F. Di Carlo

131 Concurrent Hormonal and Cytotoxic Treatment for Advanced
    Breast Cancer
    G. Robustelli Della Cuna, Q. Cuzzoni, P. Preti, and G. Bernardo

141 Hormone Dependency and Hormone Responsiveness of
    Endometrial Adenocarcinoma to Estrogens, Progestogens, and
    Antiestrogens
    J. Bonte

157 The Treatment of Endometrial Carcinoma with
    Medroxyprogesterone Acetate
    R.W. Taylor

163 A Controlled Clinical Trial on Stage I Endometrial Carcinoma:
    Rationale and Methodological Approach
    G. De Palo, C. Mangioni, P. Periti, M. Merson, and M. Del
    Vecchio

177 The Treatment of Ovarian Cancer with Medroxyprogesterone
    Acetate
    C. Bumma, O. Berbetto, and G. Gentile

183 Medroxyprogesterone Acetate in the Treatment of Prostatic Cancer:
    Preliminary Results of EORTC Trial 30761 Comparing MPA
    with Stilbestrol and with Cyproterone Acetate
    M. Pavone-Macaluso and the EORTC Urological Group

191 Medroxyprogesterone Acetate Treatment in Urological Tumors
J. Frick, R. Köhle, and H. Joos

199 Steroid Receptors and Human Renal Cell Carcinoma
F. Di Silverio and G. Concolino

211 *Subject Index*

Contributors

P. Alberto
Division of Oncology
Hospital Cantonal
1205 Geneva, Switzerland

George P. J. Alsbach
Department of Gynecology
Academic Hospital Utrecht
State University
3500 GV Utrecht, The Netherlands

H.-H. Bartsch
Department of Internal Medicine
Division of Hematology and Oncology
University of Goettingen
D-3400 Goettingen, Federal Republic of
*   Germany*

R. Battistoni
Divisione di Oncologia
Ospedale M. Malpighi
40138 Bologna, Italy

Etienne-Emile Baulieu
INSERM U 33
94270 Bicêtre, France

G. Bernardo
Division of Oncology
Clinica del Lavoro Foundation
University of Pavia
27100 Pavia, Italy

O. Bertetto
Department of Oncology
S. Giovanni Battista Hospital
10100 Turin, Italy

H.-Ch. Blossey
Department of Internal Medicine
Division of Endocrinology
University of Goettingen
D-3400 Goettingen, Federal Republic of
*   Germany*

J. Bonte
Gynecologic Cancerology
St. Rafaël Hospital
B-3000 Louvain, Belgium

C. Bumma
Department of Oncology
S. Giovanni Battista Hospital
10100 Turin, Italy

P. Burroni
Divisione di Oncologia
Ospedale M. Malpighi
40138 Bologna, Italy

C. M. Camaggi
Institute of Organic Chemistry
University of Bologna
40136 Bologna, Italy

N. Canova
Oncology Division
M. Malpighi Hospital
40138 Bologna, Italy

F. Cavalli
Division of Oncology
Ospedale San Giovanni
6500 Bellinzona, Switzerland

M. Ciuffi
Obstetrics and Gynaecology Clinic
University of Florence
50100 Florence, Italy

Giuseppe Concolino
Fifth Institute of General Clinical
*   Medicine and Therapy*
University of Rome
00161 Rome, Italy

H. Cortés Funes
Hospital "1º de Octubre"
Madrid, Spain

B. Costanti
Oncology Division
M. Malpighi Hospital
40138 Bologna, Italy

Q. Cuzzoni
Division of Oncology
Clinica del Lavoro Foundation
University of Pavia
27100 Pavia, Italy

G. De Palo
National Cancer Institute of Milan
Milan, Italy

M. Del Vecchio
National Cancer Institute of Milan
Milan, Italy

Francesco Di Carlo
Istituto di Farmacologia
University of Turin
10100 Turin, Italy

A. R. Di Marco
Divisione di Oncologia
Ospedale M. Malpighi
40138 Bologna, Italy

Franco Di Silverio
Department of Urology
Division of Urological Pathology
University of Rome
00161 Rome, Italy

Luigi Dogliotti
Clinica Medica B
University of Turin
10100 Turin, Italy

J. Frick
Urological Department
General Hospital Salzburg
Salzburg, Austria

D. Gatti
Laboratorio di Endocrinologia
  Molecolare
Università Cattolica del S. Cuore
Rome, Italy

G. Gentile
Ospedale Civile
14100 Asti, Italy

M. R. A. Gentili
Divisione di Oncologia
Ospedale M. Malpighi
40138 Bologna, Italy

M. E. Giambiasi
Divisione di Oncologia
Ospedale M. Malpighi
40138 Bologna, Italy

M. Giovannini
Divisione di Oncologia
M. Malpighi Ospedale
40138 Bologna, Italy

A. Goldhirsch
Institute for Medical Oncology
Inselspital Bern
3010 Bern, Switzerland

Inge Hesselius
Department of Gynecological Oncology
University Hospital
S-750 14 Uppsala, Sweden

S. Iacobelli
Laboratorio di Endocrinologia
  Molecolare
Università Cattolica del S. Cuore
Rome, Italy

G. Iafelice
Oncology Division
M. Malpighi Hospital
40138 Bologna, Italy

M. T. Ionta
Institute of Clinical Oncology
Cagliari Medical School
and General Cancer Hospital
09100 Cagliari, Italy

H. Joos
Urological Department
General Hospital Salzburg
Salzburg, Austria

F. Jungi
Division of Oncology
Medizinische Klinik C.
Kantonsspital St. Gallen
9006 St. Gallen, Switzerland

R. Köhle
Urological Department
General Hospital Salzburg
Salzburg, Austria

A. Lippi
Oncology Division
M. Malpighi Hospital
40138 Bologna, Italy

J. Løber
Department of Oncology A
Finsen Institute
Copenhagen, Denmark

P. L. Madrigal
Hospital Oncologico Provincial
"1º de Octubre"
Madrid, Spain

G. Perez Mangas
Hospital Oncologico Provincial
"1º de Octubre"
Madrid, Spain

C. Mangioni
I Department of Obstetrics and
    Gynecology
University of Milan
Milan, Italy

A. Martoni
Divisione di Oncologia
Ospedale M. Malpighi
40138 Bologna, Italy

G. Martz
Division of Oncology
University-Hospital
8091 Zurich, Switzerland

V. Mascia
Institute of Clinical Oncology
Cagliari Medical School
and General Cancer Hospital
09100 Cagliari, Italy

B. Massidda
Institute of Clinical Oncology
Cagliari Medical School
and General Cancer Hospital
09100 Cagliari, Italy

T. Mazzei
Department of Chemotherapy
Institute of Pharmacology and Toxicology
University of Florence
50100 Florence, Italy

C. Mendiola
Hospital "1º de Octubre"
Madrid, Spain

M. Merson
National Cancer Institute of Milan
Milan, Italy

H. T. Mouridsen
Department of Oncology A
Finsen Institute
Copenhagen, Denmark

G. Murari
Istituto di Farmacologia
Università delgi Studi di Bologna
40126 Bologna, Italy

Antonio Mussa
Clinica Chirurgica A
University of Turin
10100 Turin, Italy

G. A. Nagel
Department of Internal Medicine
Division of Hematology and Oncology
University of Goettingen
D-3400 Goettingen, Federal Republic of
    Germany

C. Natoli
Laboratorio di Endocrinologia
    Molecolare
Università Cattolica del S. Cuore
Rome, Italy

F. Pannuti
Oncology Division
M. Malpighi Hospital
40138 Bologna, Italy

M. Pavone-Macaluso
EORTC Urological Group
and Department of Urology
Polyclinic Hospital
University of Palermo School of Medicine
90127 Palermo, Italy

A. Pellegrini
Institute of Clinical Oncology
Cagliari Medical School
and General Cancer Hospital
09100 Cagliari, Italy

P. Periti
Department of Chemotherapy
Institute of Pharmacology and Toxicology
University of Florence
50100 Florence, Italy

E. Piana
Divisione di Oncologia
Ospedale M. Malpighi
40138 Bologna, Italy

P. Preti
Division of Oncology
Clinica del Lavoro Foundation
University of Pavia
27100 Pavia, Italy

G. Robustelli Della Cuna
Division of Oncology
Clinica del Lavoro Foundation
University of Pavia
27100 Pavia, Italy

C. Rose
Department of Oncology A
Finsen Institute
Copenhagen, Denmark

Derk H. Rutgers
Department of Radiotherapy
Academic Hospital Utrecht
State University
3500 GV Utrecht, The Netherlands

G. Sica
Istituo di Istologia ed Embriologia
    Generale
Università Cattolica del S. Cuore
Rome, Italy

E. Strocchi
Oncology Division
M. Malpighi Hospital
40138 Bologna, Italy

R. W. Taylor
Department of Obstetrics and
    Gynaecology
St. Thomas's Hospital Medical School
London SE1 7EH, United Kingdom

Arnold C. M. van Lindert
Department of Gynecology
Academic Hospital Utrecht
State University
3500 GV Utrecht, The Netherlands

H.-E. Wander
Department of Internal Medicine
Division of Hematology and Oncology
University of Goettingen
D-3400 Goettingen, Federal Republic of
    Germany

Role of Medroxyprogesterone in Endocrine-Related Tumors, Volume II, edited by L. Campio, G. Robustelli Della Cuna, and R. W. Taylor. Raven Press, New York © 1983.

Inhibitory Effects of Medroxyprogesterone Acetate on the Proliferation of Human Breast Cancer Cells

S. Iacobelli, *G. Sica, C. Natoli, and D. Gatti

*Laboratorio di Endocrinologia Molecolare and *Istituto di Istologia ed Embriologia Generale, Università Cattolica del S. Cuore, Rome, Italy*

Recently, a variety of hormonal agents have been introduced in the treatment of breast cancer. Medroxyprogesterone acetate (MPA) is a potent semisynthetic progestational agent that induces tumor remission in a significant number of breast cancer patients, when administered in high dosages (13,14,16). The mechanism of action of MPA and progestins in general is rather complex. MPA binds to progesterone receptors and displays antiestrogenic properties, especially on estrogen-induced stimulation of cell proliferation (11,18). It has been reported to inhibit the growth of mammary tumors in rodents and to reduce the frequency of tumor development when administered in high dosage (1). It is known that MPA exerts a negative feedback effect on the pituitary gonadal axis (3,4,15) *in vivo*, but some evidence exists that, at least in endometrial cancer *in vitro*, there is a direct cytotoxic effect on tumor cells and that specific hormone receptors are involved in this process (6,7).

Recently, it has been shown that proliferation of human breast cancer cells maintained in long-term tissue culture, such as MCF 7 cells, is inhibited by MPA (2). In this chapter we report that physiological concentrations of MPA have a direct inhibitory effect on proliferation of the CG 5 cells, a variant of the MCF 7 cell line recently obtained in our laboratory (12), and that this effect is augmented when the compound is used in association with estrogen or antiestrogen.

METHODS

CG 5 cells, a variant of the MCF 7 cell line (19), was established recently in the Laboratorio di Endocrinologia Molecolare (12). These cells contain receptors for steroid and thyroid hormones and are highly sensitive to the proliferative effect of estrogen (12). Cells were routinely cultured in Dulbecco's modified Eagle's medium supplemented with 10% fetal calf serum and antibiotics. For cell growth experiments, cells were plated out at the density of 50,000 cells/ml in medium containing 5% charcoal-treated serum. Twenty-four hours later, medium was replaced with fresh medium containing varying concentrations of compounds to be tested. In some experiments, the medium was changed every 3 days. Cells were counted after various periods of time (as specified in the text) with the use of an hemocytometer. For further details see legends of figures.

RESULTS

The addition of MPA to CG 5 cell cultures at concentrations ranging between 0.1 and 10 nM produces a dose-related inhibition of cell proliferation which reaches about 40% as compared with control cultures (Fig. 1). The extent of inhibition is not increased for hormone concentrations above 10 nM.

Figure 2 shows that a similar level of inhibition is obtained in cells exposed to estradiol plus MPA. However, under these conditions, MPA is not able to fully counteract the estrogen-stimulated cell proliferation.

If cells are cultured in the presence of varying concentrations of MPA and a fixed concentration of the antiestrogen tamoxifen, both added simultaneously at the beginning of culturing, the inhibition of cell proliferation reaches approximately 60% as compared to control cultures (Fig. 3). The inhibitory effect is already evident for MPA concentrations of 0.1 nM and it is higher than that obtained with MPA or tamoxifen alone at the same dosage (Fig. 3).

Next we examined the effects of MPA on CG 5 cells preexposed to tamoxifen. For these experiments, cells were cultured in the presence of a fixed concentration of tamoxifen for 6 days prior to the addition of MPA for 4 days. Very low doses,

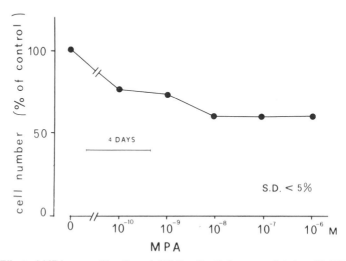

FIG. 1. Effect of MPA on proliferation of CG 5 cells. Cells were plated at 50,000 cells/ml. Twenty-four hours later medium was changed to fresh medium supplemented with 5% charcoal-treated serum and varying concentrations of MPA (from 0.1 to 1000 nM). Cells were counted 4 days after the addition of MPA. Cell number in the control plates was 700,000 cells/dish.

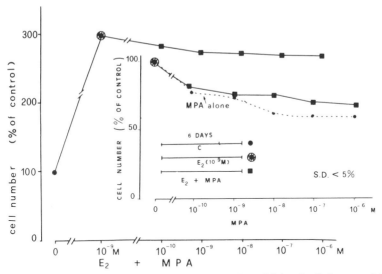

FIG. 2. Effect of estradiol and MPA added simultaneously to CG 5 cells. Cells were plated at 50,000 cells/ml. Twenty-four hours later medium was changed to fresh medium supplemented with 5% charcoal-treated serum and 1 nM estradiol or 1 nM estradiol plus varying concentrations of MPA. Cells were counted 6 days later. Cell number in control plates was 900,000 cells/dish. The *inset* also shows the effect of MPA alone.

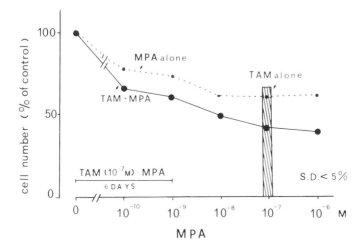

FIG. 3. Effect of tamoxifen and MPA simultaneously added to CG 5 cells. Cells were plated at 50,000 cells/ml. Twenty-four hours later medium was changed to fresh medium supplemented with charcoal-treated serum, 100 nM tamoxifen, and varying concentrations of MPA. Cells were counted 6 days later. Cell number in control plates was 636,000 cells/dish. The figure also shows the effect of tamoxifen and MPA alone.

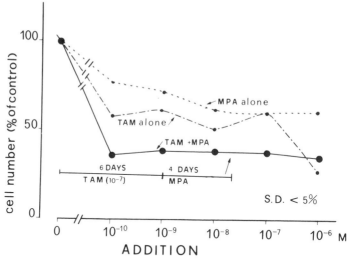

FIG. 4. Effect of tamoxifen and MPA sequentially added to CG 5 cells. Cells were plated at 50,000 cells/ml. Twenty-four hours later medium was changed to fresh medium supplemented with 5% charcoal-treated serum and 100 nM tamoxifen. After 6 days medium was changed to medium containing varying concentrations of MPA. Cells were counted 4 days later. Cell number in control plates was 800,000 cells/dish. The figure also shows the effect of tamoxifen and MPA alone.

i.e., 0.1 nM MPA, produce an inhibition of cell proliferation that reaches approximately 65% as compared to control cultures (Fig. 4).

Finally, if cells were cultured in the presence of estradiol for 6 days and then exposed to MPA in the absence of the estrogen, the inhibitory effect is very high and starts as soon as the third day after the addition of the steroid (Fig. 5). The magnitude of the inhibition reaches about 40% at physiological concentrations (0.1–10 nM) of MPA and gradually increases up to 60 and 80% after 6 and 9 days, respectively (Fig. 5).

SUMMARY

We have shown that MPA displays an inhibitory effect on the proliferation of CG 5 cells, an estrogen supersensitive variant of the MCF 7 cell line, and that this effect is higher in cells preexposed to estrogen or antiestrogen.

The reduction of cell number produced by MPA was evident at hormone concentrations in the order of 0.1–1 nM, close to the value of the dissociation constant for receptor–hormone interaction (8). This strongly suggests that the inhibitory effect of MPA on cell proliferation is mediated through a specific receptor mechanism.

McGuire and Horwitz (9) have recently demonstrated that estrogen elicits an increase of progesterone receptors in MCF 7 cells. A similar effect was produced by tamoxifen and other antiestrogenic compounds (5). Increased synthesis of progesterone receptors was recently demonstrated *in vivo* in breast cancer tissue (*this*

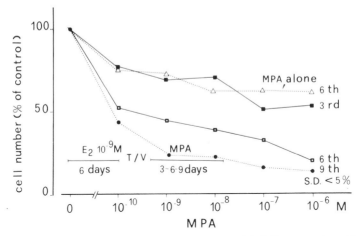

FIG. 5. Effect of MPA on CG 5 cells pretreated with estradiol. Cells were cultured for 6 days in medium supplemented with 5% charcoal-treated serum and 1 nM estradiol. At confluence, cells were trypsinized and plated at 50,000 cells/ml in medium supplemented with 5% charcoal-treated serum. Twenty-four hours later medium was changed to fresh medium supplemented with 5% charcoal-treated serum and varying concentrations of MPA. Cells were counted 3, 6, and 9 days later. On the third day cell number in control plates was 240,000 cells/dish; on the sixth day 700,000 cells/dish; on the ninth day 860,000 cells/dish.

volume, chapter 3). We have observed that CG 5 cells have a basal level of progesterone receptors of approximately 120,000 sites/cell which can be increased by about threefold after the cell's exposure to estradiol or tamoxifen (C. Natoli et al., *in preparation*). This observation explains our data showing a higher inhibitory effect of MPA in cells preexposed to either estrogen or antiestrogen as compared with unstimulated cells. Moreover, the additive effect on proliferation observed in cells exposed to MPA and tamoxifen simultaneously, higher than that seen when the two compounds are tested separately, favors the concept that these compounds act through noninteracting mechanisms.

A short comment concerns the effect of the simultaneous addition of MPA and estradiol on the proliferation of CG 5 cells. Under these conditions the stimulatory effect of estrogen is not counteracted by MPA. This has practical considerations, since it could mean that MPA might be more active in postmenopausal patients with a low level of circulating estrogens.

Finally, our data seem to warrant new trials using antiestrogens such as tamoxifen and MPA either in combination or sequentially, taking into account that they have no additive side effects, to ascertain the clinical relevance of these *in vitro* studies.

REFERENCES

1. Danguy, A., Legros, N., Devleeschouver, N., Heuson-Stennon, J.A., and Heuson, J.C. (1980): *Role of Medroxyprogesterone in Endocrine-Related Tumors*, edited by S. Iacobelli and A. Di Marco, pp. 21–28. Raven Press, New York.
2. Di Marco, A. (1980): *Role of Medroxyprogesterone in Endocrine-Related Tumors*, edited by S. Iacobelli and A. Di Marco, pp. 1–20. Raven Press, New York.

3. Ectors, F., Pasteels, J. L., and Herlant, M. (1966): *C. R. Acad. Sci. (Paris)*, 263:1988–1991.
4. Ectors, F., and Pasteels, J. L. (1967): *C. R. Acad. Sci. (Paris)*, 265:758–760.
5. Horwitz, K. B., and McGuire, W. L. (1980): *Endocrine Treatment of Breast Cancer—A New Approach*, edited by B. Henningsen, F. Linder, and C. Steichele, pp. 45–48. Springer-Verlag, Berlin, Heidelberg, New York.
6. Hustin, J. (1975): *Br. J. Obstet. Gynecol.*, 82:493–500.
7. Iacobelli, S., Longo, P., Scambia, G., Natoli, V., and Sacco, F. (1980): *Role of Medroxyprogesterone in Endocrine-Related Tumors*, edited by S. Iacobelli and A. Di Marco, pp. 97–106. Raven Press, New York.
8. King, R. B. J., and Mainwaring, W. I. P. (1974): *Steroid-Cell Interaction*. Butterworths, London.
9. McGuire, W. L., and Horwitz, K. B. (1978): *Hormones, Receptors and Breast Cancer*, edited by W. L. McGuire, pp. 31–42. Raven Press, New York.
10. Meyer, W. J., Walker, P. A., Weideking, C., Money, J., and Kowarski, A. A. (1977): *Fertil. Steril.*, 28:1072–1076.
11. Muggia, F. M., Cassileth, P. A., Ochoa, M., Jr., Flatow, F. A., Gellhorn, A., and Human, G. A. (1968): *Ann. Intern. Med.*, 68:328–337.
12. Natoli, C., Sica, G., Natoli, V., Serra, A., and Iacobelli, S.: Submitted to *Breast Cancer Research and Treatment*.
13. Pannuti, F., Freut, F., Piana, E., Strocchi, E., and Cricca, A. (1978): *IRCS Med. Sci.*, 6:118.
14. Pannuti, F., Burroni, P., Fruet, F., and Piana, E. (1979): *La Chemioterapia dei Tumori Solidi*, edited by F. Pannuti, Vol. II, pp. 805–815. Patron, Bologna.
15. Rifkind, A. B., Kulin, H. E., Cargille, C. M., Rayford, P. C., and Ross, G. T. (1969): *J. Clin. Endocrinol. Metab.*, 29:506–513.
16. Robustelli Della Cuna, G., Calciati, A., Bernardo-Strada, M. R., Bumma, C., and Campio, L. (1978): *Tumori*, 64:143–149.
17. Segaloff, A. (1966): *Recent Prog. Horm. Res.*, 22:361–379.
18. Segaloff, A., Cunningham, M., Rice, B. F., and Weeth, J. B. (1967): *Cancer*, 20:1673.
19. Soule, H. D., Vazquez, J., Long, A., Alberto, S., and Brennan, M. (1973): *J. Natl. Cancer Inst.*, 51:1409–1416.

Role of Medroxyprogesterone in Endocrine-Related Tumors, Volume II, edited by L. Campio, G. Robustelli Della Cuna, and R. W. Taylor. Raven Press, New York © 1983.

DNA Flow Cytometry of the Endometrium

Arnold C. M. van Lindert, George P. J. Alsbach, and *Derk H. Rutgers

*Department of Gynecology, Academic Hospital Utrecht, State University, 3500 GV Utrecht, The Netherlands; *Department of Radiotherapy, Academic Hospital Utrecht, State University, 3500 GV Utrecht, The Netherlands*

Cell multiplication and tissue growth is, like human endometrium, based on the concept of the cell cycle. When observing the amount of DNA per nucleus during the cell cycle, four phases can be distinguished. The G_1-phase is often the longest and in this phase the cell is prepared for DNA synthesis. The initiation of DNA synthesis makes the termination of this phase and the beginning of the S-phase. During the S-phase, DNA and other material of the chromosomes are replicated in terms of complementary strands of the Watson and Crick double helix. The amount of DNA gradually increases in the cell nucleus to the tetraploid value. After the S-phase, the cell will enter the G_2-phase. In this period, between completion of DNA synthesis and the beginning of mitosis, no changes of DNA content can be observed. In the G_2-phase the cell is preparing for the distribution of its chromosomes; the materials required for spindle formation, such as the precursors of microtubulus, are probably formed at this time. In the M-phase, which is characterized by mitosis, normally an equal distribution of the chromosomes takes place between the two daughter cells. The DNA content in each daughter cell has the diploid value.

During a normal menstrual cycle, the endometrium is continuously influenced by the growth-stimulatory effect of estrogens and the growth-inhibitory effect of progesterone. The relative distribution of cells within the synthetic phase (S-phase) and the premitotic resp. mitotic phase (G_2 + M-phase) of the cell cycle possibly reflects these phenomena. This continuous and long-lasting effect of estrogens on the endometrium often results in hyperplasia, which can be successfully treated by medroxyprogesteroneacetate (MPA). Moreover, estrogens are thought possibly to induce adenocarcinoma of the endometrium.

The aim of the present study was to establish whether or not:

a. specific patterns of the DNA-histogram can be recognized during the different phases of the menstrual cycle;

b. hyperplasia of the endometrium gives rise to unique patterns in the DNA-histogram;

c. the effect of MPA on hyperplasia of the endometrium can be monitored in the DNA-histogram;

d. adenocarcinoma of the endometrium gives rise to unique patterns in the DNA-histogram.

METHOD

The reliability of DNA measurements in endometrial cells—by means of Flow-Cytometry—largely depends on cell-processing methods such as cell-dispersion and staining of the single cell suspension. For quantitative measurement of DNA, the cell nuclei have to be stained with a fluorescent dye, which binds the cell DNA specifically and proportionally. In the present study human endometrial biopsies were obtained by abrasion. The single cell suspension was made by mincing the endometrium tissue in a Petri dish until homogeneous pulp was obtained. Further processing of the tissue fragments was done by adding 10 ml of an enzyme solution of collagenase, hyaluronidase, and pronase to the tissue fragments. The vial then was placed in a water shakebath at 34°C. The supernatant was replaced by 10 ml of the enzyme solution every 2 h. The supernatants were pooled and stored at 4°C. The cell suspension was centrifuged and fixed (methanol and acetic acid: ratio 3:1). The RNase treatment of the cells is carried out by removing the fixative followed by adding a solution with RNase and shaking in a waterbath at 34°C for 1 hr. After removal of the RNase the cells are stained for DNA with ethidium bromide. After sieving, the cell suspension was ready for fluorescence measurements in the flow cytometer (4).

Flow Cytometry and Determination of Nuclear DNA

The basic principle of flow cytometry developed by Göhde and Dittrich (2) and van Dilla (1) is the measurement of a fluorochrome, which is tagged to a specific chemical compound in the cell nucleus. In order to measure the fluorescence per single cell, the cells have to be brought into suspension and transported to a flow channel, where the individual cells pass a focused light beam. With the flow systems now available, it is possible to measure simultaneously by different cell parameters at a rate of 10^3 cells/sec. The flow cytometer system used in our measurements for relative value of DNA per cell nucleus is manufactured by Biophysics. The result of a measurement is automatically recorded in a histogram (amplitude frequency distribution) of DNA per cell, and it is possible to calculate the distribution of cells in the different phases of the cell cycle with a sophisticated computerized technique.

CLINICAL MATERIAL AND RESULTS

Endometrium and the Normal Menstrual Cycle

Endometrium biopsies from 33 women, with a strictly regular menstrual cycle of 28 days, were obtained on different days of the cycle. Only one sample per woman was taken, in order to minimize the discomfort to the woman and not to interfere with the physiological development of the uterine mucosa during the menstrual cycle.

The material was grouped in the following way:

Mid-proliferative phase:	endometrium cells obtained at cycle days 8–10
Late-proliferative phase:	" " " " " " 11–14
Early-secretory phase:	" " " " " " 15–19
Mid-secretory phase:	" " " " " " 20–24
Premenstrual phase:	" " " " " " 24–28

During the proliferative phase of a normal menstrual cycle, the median percentages of cells within S- and G_2 + M-phase of the cell cycle are 11 resp. 8. It can be judged from Fig. 1 that in the early secretory phase there is a strong and significant increase of the percentages of cells in the S-phase, which is accompanied by a decrease of the percentage of cells in the G_2 + M-phase. During the further course of the secretory phase of the menstrual cycle, the percentage of cells, both in the S-phase and G_2 + M-phase, drop to low levels.

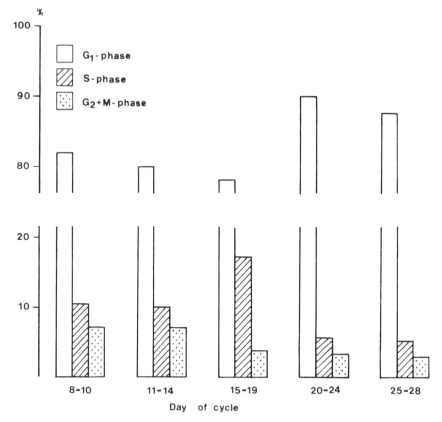

FIG. 1. This figure demonstrates the median percentages of the cells in G_1-, S-, and G_2 + M-phase of the endometrium in the different phases of the menstrual cycle.

Hyperplasia of the Endometrium

Unilateral endometrium biopsies from 14 women with histologically proved simple cystic, or adenomatous hyperplasia were taken for preparing and measuring with the flow-cytometer. Eleven women in this group were treated immediately after the unilateral biopsies with MPA, 300 mg/day per os, during 3 weeks. At the end of these weeks endometrial biopsies were taken once more for flow cytometry and from the other side of the uterus.

In the group of women with hyperplasia of the endometrium (Table 1) the average percentage of cells in the G_1-phase is 78, with a median rate of 80. Concerning the S- and G_2 + M-phase: these percentages are resp. 12 (median rate 11.5) and 10 (median rate 10). These percentages correspond with those of the endometrium in the proliferative phase. After administering MPA (Table 2) a significant decrease occurs in the average percentage of the S-phase as well as in the G_2 + M-phase, compared with the corresponding values before the treatment. The average percentage of the S-phase then is 4 (before treatment 12) and of the G_2 + M-phase 3 (before treatment 10). The average percentage in the G_1-phase increases significantly after inhibition with MPA: the average percentage then is 93 (before treatment 78).

It should be noted that in one woman with adenomatous hyperplasia no decrease occurred in the S- and the G_2 + M-phase.

Some Remarks About the Endometrium Carcinoma

Endometrium carcinomata can be subdivided histologically in well, moderately, and poorly differentiated forms. When the tumor is more poorly differentiated,

TABLE 1. *Percentages of the endometrium cells in G_1-, $S-$, and G_2+M-phase of the cell cycle of hyperplastic endometrium*

Diagnosis	G_1 (%)	S (%)	G_2+M (%)
Simple hyperplasia	56	24	20
Cystic hyperplasia	76	14	10
Simple hyperplasia	76	13	11
Cystic hyperplasia	78	9	13
Cystic hyperplasia	78	12	10
Simple hyperplasia	78	12	10
Simple hyperplasia	80	11	9
Simple hyperplasia	80	10	10
Simple hyperplasia	81	12	7
Cystic hyperplasia	81	9	10
Simple hyperplasia	81	12	7
Cystic hyperplasia	84	8	8
Adenomatous hyperplasia	84	8	8
Adenomatous hyperplasia	84	9	7
Median percentages (ultimate values in brackets)	80 (56–84)	11.5 (8–24)	10 (7–20)

TABLE 2. *MPA inhibition: Percentages of the endometrium cells in the G_1-, $S-$. and G_2+M-phase of the cell cycle of hyperplastic endometrium before and after treatment with 300 mg MPA per day during 3 to 4 weeks*

Diagnosis	Before Treatment			After Treatment		
	G_1 (%)	S (%)	G_2+M (%)	G_1 (%)	S (%)	G_2+M (%)
Simple hyperplasia	56	24	20	94	2	2
Cystic hyperplasia	76	14	10	90	6	4
Simple hyperplasia	76	13	11	94	2	4
Simple hyperplasia	80	11	9	94	3	<1
Simple hyperplasia	80	10	10	97	2	<1
Simple hyperplasia	80	12	7	92	4	4
Simple hyperplasia	81	9	10	96	3	1
Simple hyperplasia	81	12	7	93	4	3
Cystic hyperplasia	84	8	8	98	<1	<1
Adenomatous hyperplasia	84	9	7	83	10	7
Adenomatous hyperplasia	84	8	8	96	2	2
Median percentages (ultimate values in brackets)	80 (56–84)	11 (8–24)	9 (7–20)	94 (83–98)	3 (1–10)	2 (2–7)

aneuploidism of the cells is increasing. This could explain why the histogram obtained in cases of poorly differentiated tumors has a strongly aberrant aspect.

Because of such hyperaneuploidism, no clear G_2 + M-peak can be distinguished on the DNA histogram. It was not possible in these cases to calculate the percentages of cells in the different phases of the cell cycle.

Biopsies were taken from 25 women with resp. well, moderately, and poorly differentiated adenocarcinoma of the corpus uteri. Of this group, 20 women had been treated with MPA, 300 mg per day per os, during 14 to 18 days. After that, uterus and adnex extirpation followed, and biopsies were obtained for flow cytometry. It was only possible to calculate the distribution of the cells in the different phases of the cell cycle in 3 cases out of the 13 women with an untreated, poorly differentiated adenocarcinoma of the endometrium. In the case of 12 women with well to moderately differentiated carcinomas, the DNA histogram of the tumors was justified in only 8 cases to calculate the G_1-, S-, and G_2 + M-phase, according to our method. In two cases of 8 women treated with MPA, it was possible to calculate the percentages of G_1-, S-, and G_2 + M-phase of the DNA-histogram.

In Table 3 the percentages of the G_1-, S-, and G_2 + M-phase of the untreated group are reproduced. The average percentages of the G_1-, S-, and G_2 + M-phase are resp. 83 (median rate 82), 8 (median rate 8), 9 (median rate 9). These average rates do not deviate much from the percentages for proliferative and hyperplastic endometrium. In only two cases the histogram could be used both before and after the treatment with MPA, 300 mg per day per os, during resp. 15 and 17 days.

TABLE 3. *Adenocarcinoma of the endometrium: Percentages of endometrium cells in the G_1-, $S-$, and G_2+M-phase of the cell cycle of endometrium carcinoma*

Histologic Differentiation	G_1 (%)	S (%)	G_2+M (%)
Well differentiated	91	4	5
Well differentiated	91	6	3
Well differentiated	85	6	9
Well differentiated	84	8	8
Well differentiated	82	10	8
Well differentiated	79	11	10
Well differentiated	76	11	13
Moderately differentiated	74	13	13
Poorly differentiated	87	7	6
Poorly differentiated	82	8	10
Poorly differentiated	81	9	9
Median percentages (ultimate values in brackets)	82 (74–91)	8 (4–13)	9 (3–13)

TABLE 4. *Effect of MPA on endometrium carcinoma of two patients*

Diagnosis	Before Treatment			After Treatment		
	G_1 (%)	S (%)	G_2+M (%)	G_1 (%)	S (%)	G_2+M (%)
Well differentiated adenocarcinoma	82	10	8	94	5	1
Moderately differentiated adenocarcinoma	74	13	13	90	6	4

From Table 4 the conclusion can be drawn that a significant decrease of the percentage of cells in the S_1- and G_2 + M-phase has taken place.

DISCUSSION

The results obtained with the DNA-flow-cytometry demonstrate a variation of the cell kinetic pattern of human endometrium during a normal menstrual cycle. This also counts for hyperplastic endometrium and the effect of MPA. Because of the difficulties that were partly of a preparative and partly of a mathematical nature, this could not be proved for the endometrium carcinoma. In the mid-proliferative phase of a menstrual cycle a clear activity of DNA synthesis of endometrium cells is present, compared with the mid-secretory phase and the premenstrual phase, according to the raised percentages of cells in the S-phase and the G_2 + M-phase, resp. 11 and 7.5 (median rates). This pattern continues in the late proliferative phase which corresponds to the autoradiographic notes of others.

In our present study, a significant increase of cells in the S-phase is observed during the early secretory phase; however, there is a significant decrease of cells in the G_2 + M-phase of the cell-cycle, compared with the number of cells in the proliferative phase. This increase of the percentage of cells in the S-phase in the early-secretory phase can be explained by assuming that under the influence of increasing progesterone levels in the beginning of the second half of the menstrual cycle an increasing inhibition of the cells in the S-phase is present beginning in the late S-phase. Probably the decrease of the G_2 + M-phase has been caused by the decreased transit of cells from the S-phase to the G_2 + M-phase under the influence of progesterone.

A prolongation of the S-phase in the early secretory phase, as compared with that in the proliferative phase, is correlated to a decrease of tritium thymidine uptake per time unit of these cells in the S-phase. A decrease of the tritium thymidine uptake of endometrium cells in this period of the menstrual cycle was noticed by Nordqvist (3). Noticeable is a significant decrease of cells in the S-phase during the mid-secretory phase; this compared to the number of cells during the proliferative phase and the early secretory phase. The amount of cells in the G_2 + M-phase, during the mid-secretory phase, continues to be on the same level as during the early secretory phase.

It is possible that long-lasting progesterone stress causes a decrease of the growth fraction of the endometrium cells. There is some evidence from Japanese studies with autoradiographic techniques that progesterone inhibits the estrogen-induced proiferation of the endometrium cells in the early G_1-phase of the cell cycle and will transfer the cycle cells to the resting stage, the G_0-stage.

In our study the premenstrual phase shows no difference from the secretory phase. The kinetic patterns of hyperplastic endometrium are equal to those of the proliferative phase of the normal menstrual cycle. After treatment with MPA, 300 mg per day per os during 3 to 4 weeks, a significant decrease of the percentages of cells in the S- and G_2 + M-phase does occur. Because of this uniform effect of MPA in cases of hyperplasia of the endometrium, the DNA flow cytometry makes it possible to fix the optimal dose of this hormone for regression of the endometrium.

REFERENCES

1. Dilla, M. A. van, Trujillo, T. T., Mullaney, P. F., and Coulter, J. R. (1969): *Science*, 163:1213.
2. Dittrich, W., and Göhde (1969): *Z. Naturforsch.*, 246:360.
3. Nordqvist, S. (1970): *J. Endocrinol.*, 48:17.
4. Rutgers, D. H. (1980): Cell preparation of solid tumors for flow cytometry. *Acta Pathol. Microbiol. Scand. (in press)*.

Role of Medroxyprogesterone in Endocrine-Related Tumors, Volume II, edited by L. Campio, G. Robustelli Della Cuna, and R. W. Taylor. Raven Press, New York © 1983.

A Rationale for Combined Antiestrogen plus Progestin Administration in Breast Cancer

Etienne-Emile Baulieu

Inserm U 33, 94270 Bicêtre, France

In more than two-thirds of breast cancers (unselected cases), estradiol receptor (ER) is found in concentration believed to be sufficient for mediating estrogen action. These cases are "ER + ." It is known that most tumors are heterogeneous in terms of receptor-containing cells, and that ER is a necessary but not sufficient cellular component for obtaining a response to estrogens or antiestrogens. In fact, ~50% of patients whose tumors are ER + (>20 fmol/mg cytosol protein) respond to hormonal manipulation (2,7). By far these ER + responsive cancers are those that contain, in addition, progesterone receptor (PR + >20 fmol/mg cytosol protein) (1,8), a marker of estrogen action (9) (~30% of cancers are ER + , PR + , and 80% of those cases are responsive to hormonal therapy). However, not only do some ER + , PR + cases not respond to endocrine treatments, but more interestingly ~30–40% of ER + , PR − tumors are responsive. We have proposed a "hormonal challenge test" (13) which may be able to detect early such patients likely to benefit from appropriate adjunctive hormonal therapy. The test is based on the ER-dependent PR increase provoked by the antiestrogen tamoxifen.

HORMONAL CHALLENGE TEST WITH TAMOXIFEN

Tamoxifen is an antiestrogen showing a significant effect on the division and growth of estrogen target cells, not only in avian (21) but also in mammalian species (3). It binds to ER, occupying estradiol binding sites. Wherever the receptor is localized in the cytoplasmic or in the nuclear compartment of estradiol target cells, there is formation of antiestrogen–receptor complexes in as much as the concentration of the antiestrogen and its relative affinity for the receptor are appropriate to compete with estradiol. These antiestrogen–receptor complexes do not promote the division of target cells, like estrogen–receptor complexes. However, in several instances, they are responsible for the synthesis of specific proteins, in particular that of PR. Such "dissociated" effect, with absence of estrogen-like action on cell multiplication and estrogen-like positive effect on specific protein synthesis, in particular PR, make tamoxifen an interesting drug for challenging the estrogen responsive machinery of cancer cells, without risk of stimulation of tumor growth.

The hormonal challenge test with tamoxifen consists of measuring PR in tumor samples before and after administration of the drug. The increase in PR concentration indicates a potential for these patients to benefit from hormonal therapy.

In a small number of breast cancer patients with cutaneous metastases (13), tamoxifen (30 mg × 7 days) displayed properties predictable from laboratory animal and *in vitro* experiments. No ER − tumors showed a response. Approximately 50% of the ER + cases did not respond, including some cases originally with PR + . As expected (1), most ER + , PR − cancers did not respond, but there was a definitive increase of PR in one case. As in endometrial cancer (10,17), it appears that a dynamic test may be more valuable than a single set of receptor measurements in assessing hormone sensitivity of breast carcinoma.

In animal experiments, tamoxifen binds to ER in the cytoplasm, and the tamoxifen–ER complexes migrate to the nucleus, resulting in a decrease of the cytoplasmic receptor concentration. The latter finding was observed in all ER + breast cancer samples after tamoxifen administration, indicating that tamoxifen had reached its target cells. Whether this decrease is only due to transfer of the tamoxifen–ER complexes to the nucleus, or also to the diminution of the total ER concentration following a week of antiestrogen treatment is not known, since ER had not been measured in the nuclear fraction. In any event our preliminary results have been confirmed (16). The use of needle biopsies (drill), combined with appropriate miniaturization of the technique of receptor determination (4,5), should make possible the use of the hormonal challenge test in other metastases and in the primary tumor itself, even at an early stage of the disease.

COMBINED ADMINISTRATION OF ANTIESTROGEN AND PROGESTIN

We have suggested that, in addition to the predictive value of the challenge test, and besides the proper antiestrogen effect of tamoxifen (6,11), the utilization of this agent may also be viewed as a potential primer for progestin action.

Progestin treatment of breast cancer is not new. Many authors have reported on the antiestrogenic properties of progesterone, especially on estrogen-stimulated growth (12,18–20). However, the administration of "low" doses of progestin, in the order of $< \sim 100$ mg/day, appears to be the least efficient hormonal treatment of breast cancer. Recently Pannuti and several others (14; *this volume*) have successively

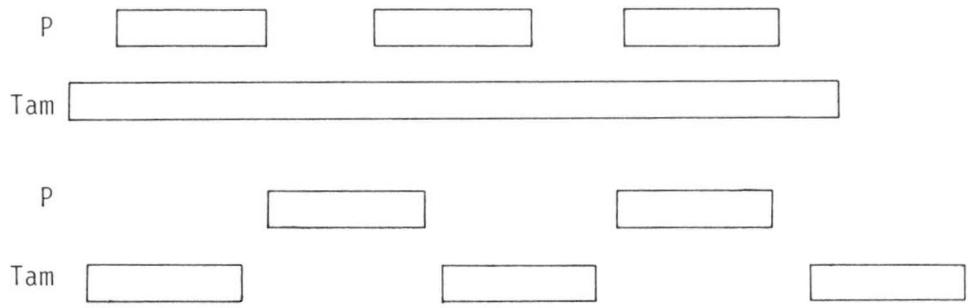

FIG. 1.   Rectangles indicate a period of treatment. Small rectangles may be 4 to 15 days long.

used much larger doses of medroxyprogesterone acetate (MPA), and obtained results comparable to other active hormonal therapy, i.e., tamoxifen and aminogluthetimide (a suppressor of steroid biosynthesis). Even if only minimal side effects have yet been reported, administration of 1 gm/day and of even larger doses *(this volume)* of a steroid for several weeks may not be justified. Unforeseen difficulties may occur, related in particular to the known effects of large doses of progesterone in the CNS (15).

The determination of progesterone action is rather complex. Besides a direct effect on breast cancer cells, negative feedback mechanism on pituitary function and general anabolic activity may be important. These effects are either totally or partly mediated by receptor mechanisms, i.e., the PR (for breast, hypothalamic, and pituitary cells), and possibly by the androgen and the glucocorticosteroid receptors for the poorly defined anabolic activity. However, we wonder what could be the consequences of the several hundreds ng/ml concentration of progestin established in the plasma during high dose administration. Are there unknown beneficial specific mechanisms or is it only a manner to compensate the low PR concentration, decreased by the treatment by progestin itself as in the uterus (9), according to the law of mass action:

$$\text{size of progestin effect : f (progestin) (PR).}$$

This "equation" indicates that, for a given hormone concentration, within certain limits, the receptor concentration is critical. Likewise, for a given receptor concentration, within certain limits, the concentration of hormone is critical.

It is therefore more promising in our opinion to try to rescue the PR concentration, therefore rendering the cells potentially more responsive to progestin. Hopefully it then would be sufficient to establish progestin concentrations nearer to physiological levels, in contrast to the presently proposed administration of very high doses of MPA.

Efficient schedule and dose of antiestrogen and progestin administrations are yet to be established. Some investigators (Pellegrini et al., *this volume*) are even still proposing the use of an estrogen (ethinylestradiol) rather than antiestrogen as a primer for progesterone action, in order to increase the number of cells entering cell division cycle and promote progesterone action (Periti et al., *this volume*). In view of mitogenic effect of estrogens, we prefer antiestrogen, since it appears as active as estrogen in the rescue of PR. It remains to be established, however, whether simultaneous is preferable to the sequential administration of antiestrogen and progestin. We favor the discontinuous schedule, since the aim is to overcome the negative progesterone effect on its receptor concentration (9). Among the possibilities, one can consider either alternate administration of tamoxifen and progestin for each 4- to 15-day period, or continuous administration of tamoxifen with progestin given every 4–15 days (Fig. 1).

Interrupting both hormonal treatments for a few days from time to time can also be proposed to use possible rebound phenomenon prior to further courses of treatment. In any case, the pharmacokinetic particularities of antiestrogen and progestin should always be considered, and in particular the prolonged action of tamoxifen and of intramuscularly administered progestin.

REFERENCES

1. Horwitz, K. B., McGuire, W. L., Pearson, O. H., and Segaloff, A. (1975): *Science*, 189:726–727.
2. Jensen, E. V., DeSombre, E. R., and Jungblut, P. W. (1967): *Endogenous Factors Influencing Host Tumor Balance*, edited by R. W. Wissler, T. L. Dao, and S. Wood, pp. 15–30. University of Chicago Press, Chicago.
3. Jordan, V. C., Dix, C. J., Naylor, K. E., Prestwich, G., and Roswsby, L. (1978): *J. Toxicol. Environ. Health*, 4:363–390.
4. Magdelénat, H. (1979): *Cancer Treat. Rep.*, 63:1146.
5. Magdelénat, H., Toubeau, M., Picco, C., and Bidron, C. (1981): *Récepteurs Hormonaux et Pathologie Mammaire*, edited by P. M. Martin, pp. 107–119. Medsi, Paris.
6. Manni, A., Trujillo, J. E., Marshall, J. S., Brodkey, J., and Pearson, O. H. (1979): *Cancer*, 43:444–450.
7. McGuire, W. L., Carbone, P. P., and Vollmer, E. P., editors (1975): *Estrogen Receptors in Human Breast Cancer*, Raven Press, New York.
8. McGuire, W. L., Raynaud, J. P., and Baulieu, E. E., editors (1977): *Progesterone Receptors in Normal and Neoplastic Tissues*, Raven Press, New York.
9. Milgrom, E., Luu Thi, M., Atger, M., and Baulieu, E. E. (1973): *J. Biol. Chem.*, 248:6366–6374.
10. Mortel, R., Levy, C., Wolff, J. P., Nicolas, J. C., Robel, P., and Baulieu, E. E. (1981): *Cancer Res.*, 41:1140–1147.
11. Mouridsen, H., Palshof, T., Patterson, J., and Battersby, L. (1978): *Cancer Treat. Rev.*, 5:131–141.
12. Muggia, F. M., Cassileth, P. A., Ochoa, M., Jr., Flatow, F. A., Gellhorn, A., and Human, G. A. (1968): *Ann. Intern. Med.*, 68:328–337.
13. Namer, M., Lalanne, C., and Baulieu, E. E. (1980): *Cancer Res.*, 40:1750–1752.
14. Pannuti, F., Di Marco, A. R., Martoni, A., Fruet, F., Strocchi, E., Burroni, P., Rossi, A. P., and Cricca, A. (1980): *Role of Medroxyprogesterone in Endocrine-Related Tumors*. In: *Progress in Cancer Research and Therapy, Vol. 15*, edited by S. Iacobelli and A. Di Marco, pp. 73–92. Raven Press, New York.
15. Phillipps, G. H. (1974): *Molecular Mechanisms in General Anaesthesia*, edited by M. J. Massley, R. A. Millar, and J. A. Sutton, pp. 32–47. Churchill-Livingstone, London.
16. Pouillard, P., Palamgié, T., Jouve, M., Garcia-Girald, E., and Magdelénat, H. (1981): *Presse Médicale (in press)*.
17. Robel, P., Levy, C., Wolff, J. P., Nicolas, J. C., and Baulieu, E. E. (1978): *C. R. Hebd. Séances Acad. Sci.*, 287:1353–1356.
18. Rubens, R. D., Knight, R. K., and Hayward, J. L. (1976): *Eur. J. Cancer*, 12:563–565.
19. Segaloff, A., Cuningham, M., Rice, B. F., and Weeth, J. B. (1967): *Cancer*, 20:1673.
20. Stoll, A. (1967): *Br. Med. J.*, 3:338.
21. Sutherland, R. L., Mester, J., and Baulieu, E. E. (1977): *Nature*, 267:434–453.

Role of Medroxyprogesterone in Endocrine-Related Tumors, Volume II, edited by L. Campio, G. Robustelli Della Cuna, and R. W. Taylor. Raven Press, New York © 1983.

Pharmacokinetics of Oral Medroxyprogesterone Acetate at Moderate Doses in a Long-Term Study

*P. Periti, **M. Ciuffi, and *T. Mazzei

*Department of Chemotherapy, Institute of Pharmacology and Toxicology, and **Obstetrics and Gynaecology Clinic; University of Florence, 50100 Florence, Italy

Clinical pharmacology clearly has an important role in the use of antineoplastic agents. Comprehensive analysis conducted at the time of initial clinical trial with the primary goals of defining the absorption, distribution, elimination, and metabolism of a drug is desirable with the ultimate aim of achieving an optimal clinical schedule and dose. Only recently, with the development of new technological advances, has this become possible, and therefore many of the commonly used antineoplastic drugs are only now being clearly defined as to their pharmacokinetic behavior. Recent years have witnessed a definite increase in reliable clinical pharmacology in medical oncology, suggesting a more specific role for routine drug level monitoring to improve either the safety or efficacy of antineoplastic chemotherapy (1).

Routine drug monitoring may allow dose adjustment on a more rational basis than is presently used; moreover, for drugs having a prolonged plasma half-life, patient compliance can be verified by blood level assay.

Wide fluctuations in drug absorption, metabolism, or elimination may be responsible for intra-individual variation in pharmacokinetics and the inconstant manifestations of clinical toxicity. The same factors may lead to considerable variability in effectiveness of fixed doses of routine clinical use. Therefore, the value of pharmacokinetic data depends on the identification during comprehensive studies of a single time point reflecting the intra-individual variation that may result in increased toxicity or a compromise of therapeutic effect. However, the neoplastic process is heterogeneous and this heterogenicity may complicate the correlation of therapeutic effect with classic pharmacokinetic parameters such as plasma drug concentration; moreover, prediction of efficacy and safety on the basis of drug levels presupposes that changes in plasma reflect those within target tissues, and final evaluation will probably require an integrative approach of pharmacokinetics, biochemical pharmacology, and cell kinetics. A particular instance in which pharmacokinetics may have a role in the clinical use of an anticancer drug is perhaps

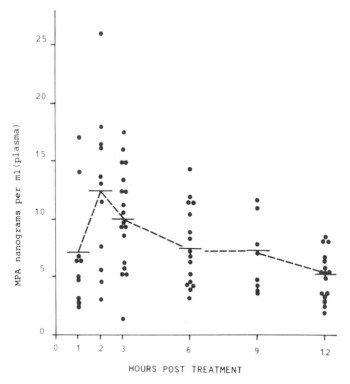

FIG. 1. Plasma concentration of MPA in women who received 100 mg single oral dose (*dotted line*, mean; *circles*, plasma MPA measurement: RIA method).

suggested by recent studies on moderate or high dose medroxyprogesterone acetate (MPA) in a long-term treatment by intramuscular or oral route (3,4).

Since February 1980 we have been involved in a national protocol of adjuvant hormonal therapy for endometrial carcinoma at Stage I disease employing MPA orally for 12 months. There are very few reports on blood levels of MPA in the human and consequently it was decided to monitor the drug during treatment. This report is concerned with the pilot pharmacokinetic study done during the follow-up of a group of women who had undergone surgical therapy for endometrial adenocarcinoma and adjuvant treatment with oral MPA.

MATERIAL AND METHODS

A group of 22 patients affected by endometrial cancer (Stage I) were treated after surgery with 100 mg twice daily of oral MPA for 12 months; the interval between every dose was 12 h. The plasma measurements were made over a 12-hr period after administration of the first 100 mg tablet (Farlutal®) or before giving the morning dose throughout the 1 year of treatment, and at random from the first to the twelfth month. Venous blood samples were withdrawn into heparinized tubes and the plasma

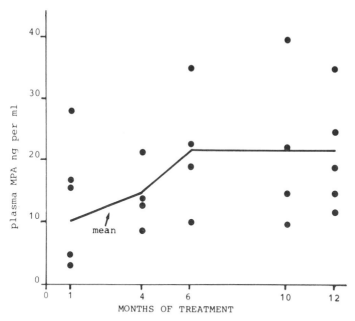

FIG. 2. Routine MPA plasma monitoring during 12 months of adjuvant therapy for endometrial cancer (MPA 2 × 100 mg every 12 hr orally). Plasma samples were taken before giving the morning dose (*circles*, plasma MPA measurement; RIA method).

separated by centrifugation and stored at −20°C until analyzed. Plasma MPA was determined by radioimmunoassay method, utilizing an antiserum against MPA-3-(O-carboxymethyl) oxime-BSA provided by the Upjohn Company, USA; 1.2-³H-MPA obtained from the New England Nuclear Company with specific activity of 60 Ci/mmole was used as tracer (5). The antiserum has a substantial cross-reaction with metabolites of MPA: there is no reaction with naturally occurring steroids.

In 4 cases we compared the bio-availability of MPA from two commercial sources in tablets containing 100 mg of the steroid as Provera® (Upjohn) or Farlutal® (Farmitalia), crossing the two pharmaceutical preparations with an interval of 2 days in every case and determining the plasma MPA levels over 12 hr after the administration of each tablet.

RESULTS

The results of this study are presented in Figs. 1–4. In Fig. 1 are reported data on plasma MPA levels in 18 patients over 12 hr after oral administration of 100 mg as a single dose: a maximum mean concentration of 12.4 ng/ml was reached in the blood at the second hour and it was followed by a decline curve with a half-life of 8.66 hours ($y = 2.6 − 0.07\ x$). The MPA level measurable at 12 hr, that is, just before administration of the next dose, is the time point reflecting the intra-individual variation and is useful in routine monitoring of the drug; after the first

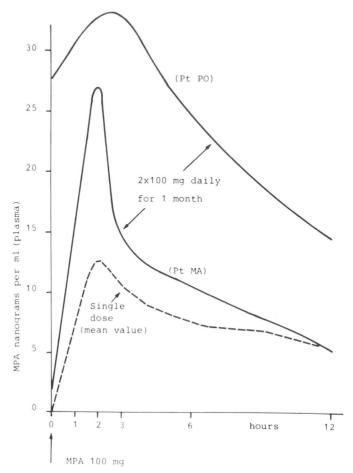

FIG. 3. Plasma concentrations of MPA in 2 patients who received MPA orally 2 × 100 mg daily for 1 month. Comparison with plasma level after single MPA 100 mg oral dose (see Fig. 1).

dose this level corresponds to a mean value of 5.17 ng/ml with a range between 2 and 8.4 ng/ml.

The trough of MPA disappearance in plasma is chosen as a valid reflection of the drug's pharmacokinetic behavior for routine monitoring in a long-term therapy.

In Fig. 2 the single time point behavior at different months of treatment for groups of 4–5 patients is shown: The trough's mean values are increasing in the first 6 months from 10 to 20 ng/ml and a steady state on this level is then maintined till the end of the treatment. Since MPA has prolonged plasma half-life we can suppose that there is a peak two to three times higher than the trough, and that the blood concentrations between the 100-mg doses must rise to very high levels of about 30–50 ng/ml and fall to 10–20 ng/ml twice a day every 12 hr.

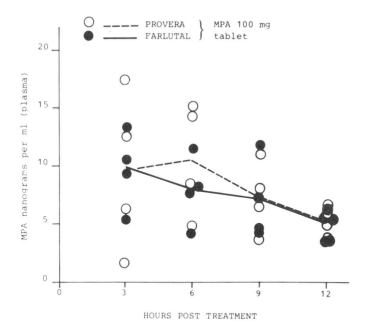

HOURS POST TREATMENT

FIG. 4. Plasma levels comparison in 4 patients who received at the start of MPA treatment a 100-mg oral dose as tablet of Provera® or Farlutal® in a crossed administration to the same subject with 4 days interval between the different commercial preparations [plasma MPA measurements and mean values after Provera® (*open circles* and *dotted lines*) or Farlutal® (*closed circles* and *solid lines*): RIA method].

These fluctuations correspond to molar concentrations of approximately 10^{-7}–10^{-8} M. Levels such as this *in vitro* have a marked cytoreductive effect on endometrial cancer cells and *in vivo* are capable of a marked progestational activity (2).

As an example of the role of routine drug plasma level monitoring during MPA oral long-term therapy, we show in Fig. 3 the different steroid pharmacokinetics in 2 patients at the end of the first month in comparison with the behavior after a single 100-mg dose at the start of the treatment. It is evident that the validity of the single time point chosen, corresponding to the trough for the identification of intra-individual variations in plasma mpa levels, may perhaps result at the end of our clinical controlled study of a predictive value for the safety and the efficacy of the adjuvant hormonal therapy.

In Fig. 4 are reported the data concerning the comparison of plasma levels after oral administration with 2 days interval to the same patients of MPA, 100 mg as a Provera® or Farlutal® tablet. There is no difference in the mean values over the 12 hr after each administration.

Urine samples taken at random during MPA oral therapy in 5 patients have shown a low concentration with a mean value of 15 ng/ml (range 4.2–25.0).

CONCLUSIONS

1. Oral MPA at 100 mg dose every 12 hr can assure plasma concentrations between 10^{-8} and 10^{-7} M in all patients treated by the oral route.

2. The steady state of plasma levels is reached after the fourth month of daily treatment with oral 2×100 mg MPA.

3. The single time point for routine MPA monitoring corresponds to the trough of the curve of drug disappearance in plasma and is a valid reflection of the drug's pharmacokinetic behavior in each patient.

4. Routine MPA monitoring could be helpful in prediction of therapeutic or toxic effects during a long-term treatment because the intra-individual pharmacokinetic variations are substantial.

5. Further investigation is indicated on plasma MPA levels routinely monitored not only during hormonal adjuvant therapy but especially in coincidence of palliative treatment of advanced or recurrent endometrial adenocarcinoma with the aim of a possible correlation of pharmacokinetics to the clinical efficacy of the drug.

ACKNOWLEDGMENT

This work was supported by CNR Grant, contract no. 81.01435.96, Subproject "Combined Therapy", of the Project "Control of Neoplastic Growth", National Research Council.

REFERENCES

1. Erlichman, C., Donehower, R. C., and Chabner, B. A. (1980): *Cancer Chemother. Pharmacol.*, 4:139–145.
2. Iacobelli, S., Longo, P., Scambia, G., Natoli, V., and Sacco, F. (1980): *Role of Medroxyprogesterone in Endocrine-Related Tumors*, edited by S. Iacobelli and A. Di Marco, pp. 97–106. Raven Press, New York.
3. Laatikainen, T., Nieminen, U., and Adlercreutz, H. (1979): *Acta Obstet. Gynecol. Scand.*, 58:95–99.
4. Salimtschik, M., Mouridsen, H. T., Loeber, J., and Johansson, E. (1980): *Cancer Chemother. Pharmacol.*, 4:267–269.
5. Shrimanker, K., Saxena, B. N., and Fotherby, K. (1978): *J. Steroids Chemistry*, 9:359–363.

Role of Medroxyprogesterone in Endocrine-Related Tumors, Volume II, edited by L. Campio, G. Robustelli Della Cuna, and R. W. Taylor. Raven Press, New York © 1983.

Pharmacokinetics of Medroxyprogesterone Acetate and Plasma Levels in a Long-Term Treatment

Inge Hesselius

Department of Gynecological Oncology, University Hospital, S-750 14 Uppsala, Sweden

Medroxyprogesterone acetate (17-alpha-acetoxy-6-alpha-methyl-4-pregnene-3,20 dione, MPA) was first synthesized in 1958 (2,11) and has been widely used ever since for the treatment of advanced endometrial carcinoma, in which progestins have been reported to cause regression of tumor growth in a considerable proportion of cases (1,3). The MPA doses were and in some places still are moderate, 250–300 mg intramuscularly once a week (12). However, as proposed by Bonte (3) among others several clinics began to administer 1000 mg MPA intramuscularly once weekly.

With the introduction of MPA tablets, the question arose of giving equipotent doses of MPA via the intramuscular versus the oral route. As there were so few reports on blood levels of MPA and these dealt with lower doses for contraceptive purposes (5,10), it was decided to measure the plasma levels of MPA in patients with endometrial carcinoma following either intramuscular or oral administration of MPA. A study was designed to investigate the pharmacokinetics of MPA in different individuals on different dosages via oral or intramuscular administration. As the plasma levels following an initial single dose of MPA administered orally or intramuscularly could not be expected to reflect the plasma levels throughout a life-long treatment period, a long-term study was designed to compare oral vis-a-vis intramuscular administration of MPA. Thus the problem of equipotent doses could be elucidated (7).

In the treatment of advanced breast cancer high daily doses of 500–1000 mg MPA are used in several clinics. Such high doses of MPA are either administered orally in daily doses in a continuous treatment scheme or intramuscularly in daily doses during a loading phase followed by weekly doses in the maintenance phase of the treatment.

For an adequate evaluation of the clinical results obtained with such different treatment models a comparison of blood levels of MPA is necessary.

25

MATERIAL AND METHODS

Patients

In 15 patients with endometrial carcinoma, progestin treatment was introduced by administering intramuscularly 1000 mg MPA. Blood samples were taken prior to injection and then after 1, 2, 4, 6, 8, 12, 24, 28, 32, 36, 48, 60, and 72 hr. In another group of 9 patients, MPA as a single dose of 100 mg was administered orally and blood samples were taken prior to ingestion of MPA and then after every hour for 6 hr. In a third group, 12 patients were given 200 mg MPA as a single oral dose and blood samples were taken at 0, 1, 2, 4, 6, 8, 24, 32, 48, 56, and 72 hr. Two other groups of 4 patients each received MPA as a single intramuscular dose, 500 mg and 1000 mg, respectively. Blood samples were drawn prior to the MPA dose and then daily for 14 days.

A total of 30 patients were divided into groups of 10, each of which was to be treated with a different dosage scheme. Patients with a very poor prognosis and not expected to live more than a few months had to be excluded from the trial. Each patient accepted into the trial was randomly allocated to one of three treatment groups:

1. MPA 1000 mg intramuscularly once a week;
2. MPA 1000 mg intramuscularly once every 2 weeks; and
3. MPA 100 mg orally twice daily.

Blood was drawn from each patient prior to starting treatment with MPA. For patients in groups 1 and 2, blood was taken once every 4 weeks immediately before the next injection. For patients in group 3, blood was also drawn once every 4 weeks, if possible before the morning dose of MPA; in other cases, just before the second MPA dose of the day. This procedure was pursued for 52 weeks for all the three groups. In addition, at 12 weeks, blood was taken prior to the MPA dose and then hourly for 6 hours in (a) 7 patients in the group given 1000 mg MPA once a week, and (b) 8 patients on 100 mg MPA twice daily in oral doses. Five patients were given daily oral MPA doses of 1000 mg (400 mg at 8 A.M. and 600 mg at 8 P.M.). Blood samples were drawn before the morning dose after 7, 14, and 21 days of MPA treatment.

A group of 11 patients was treated with daily intramuscular injections of 1000 mg MPA for 14 days. Blood samples were taken 24 hr after the seventh and fourteenth injections. This loading dose of 1000 mg MPA daily for 14 days was followed by a maintenance dose of 1000 mg MPA weekly. In 4 patients blood samples were taken 24 hr after the MPA injections after 7, 14, 21, and 28 days of treatment. In this way two different dosage schemes are compared in Figs. 11 and 12.

Radioimmunologic Method

MPA was measured by radioimmunoassay using an antiserum prepared by Cornette et al. (4). The antigen was prepared by coupling MPA at the 3-position to bovine serum albumin. The antiserum was provided by Upjohn Co., Kalamazoo, MI, as was the crystalline MPA used as a standard. H^3-1,2-medroxyprogesterone acetate, with a specific activity of 58 Ci/mmol was purchased from New England Nuclear Corporation and used as tracer in the assay. The serum samples were extracted once by petroleum ether prior to radioimmunoassay (7,13).

RESULTS

A single dose of 1000 mg MPA administered intramuscularly does not produce peak values in the blood levels of MPA. After 8–12 hr a level of 10–15 ng/ml was reached and this was maintained throughout the 72 hr studied (Fig. 1). This figure represents the mean MPA level of 15 women. There were considerable interindividual differences in plasma levels which cannot be correlated to differences in body weight or body surface area. The plateau values obtained were maintained throughout a 14-day period (Fig. 2). Due to considerable interindividual differences, with extremely low values in one of the 4 patients studied, the mean values in the 1000 mg groups are lower than shown in Fig. 1. A linear correlation between administered dose and blood levels of MPA is illustrated.

Ingestion of a single oral dose of 100 mg MPA in a group of 9 patients gave mean plasma levels with a fast absorption and distribution phase and a peak value of above 10 ng/ml. A fast elimination phase results in a mean plasma value of about 40% of the peak value after 6 hr (Fig. 3). A single oral dose of 200 mg MPA gives a similar curve (Fig. 4).

From a mean peak value of nearly 15 ng/ml a fast breakdown of MPA results in levels of 28 and 19% of the peak values after 8 and 24 hr, respectively. The interindividual differences are still more pronounced after the oral administration

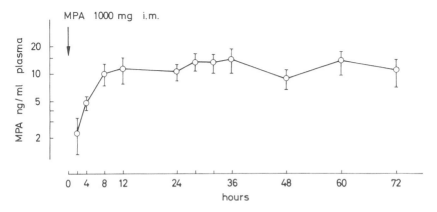

FIG. 1. Plasma concentrations of MPA after i.m. administration of a single dose of 1000 mg MPA to 15 patients. Mean ± SEM.

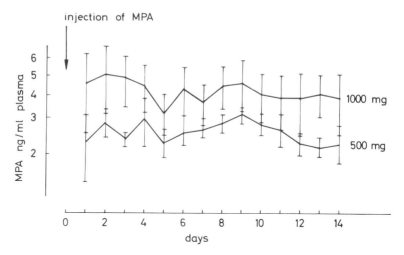

FIG. 2. Plasma concentrations of MPA after i.m. administration of single doses of 500 mg to 4 patients and 1000 mg MPA to another group of 4 patients. Mean ± SEM.

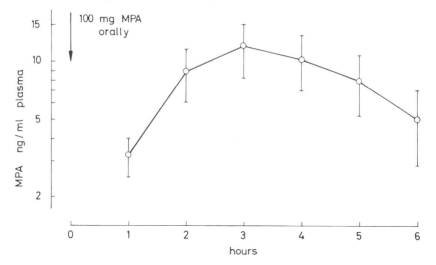

FIG. 3. Plasma concentrations of MPA after oral administration of a single dose of 100 mg MPA to 9 patients. Mean ± SEM.

of MPA, but even in this case, no correlation could be found between the MPA dose and body weight or body surface. The interindividual differences were most pronounced in the 100 mg group of 9 women with advanced cancer in comparison with the 200 mg group in which MPA was given as adjuvant therapy to patients with an excellent performance status.

When administered intramuscularly once a week, MPA was found to cause steadily increasing plasma levels, whereas the daily oral doses led to a steady state.

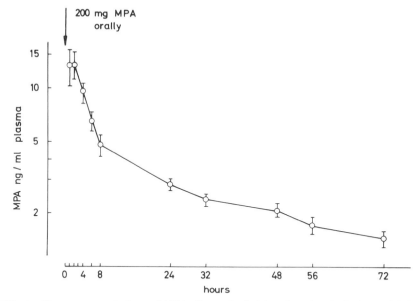

FIG. 4. Plasma concentrations of MPA after oral administration of a single dose of 200 mg MPA to 12 women. Mean ± SEM.

After a treatment period of 12 weeks the mean plasma levels were significantly higher in a group in which MPA was administered intramuscularly in comparison with another group on oral MPA dosage.

Therefore, to complete the pharmacokinetic study the effects of a MPA dose after 12 weeks' treatment with the two different regimens are presented (Figs. 5 and 6). From a base level of 12.1 ng/ml an oral dose of 100 mg MPA gave a mean peak value of 23.6 ng/ml in 8 patients (Fig. 5).

The intramuscular injection in 7 patients of a new weekly dose of 1000 mg MPA (Fig. 6) produced a slightly rising curve for the mean plasma levels, from a mean base value of 43.7 ng/ml to a mean peak value of 57.7 ng/ml. Thus, even when the higher peak values with the oral administration are considered the MPA plasma levels are significantly higher in the intramuscular group.

In the long-term plasma level study of three different MPA treatment regimens there was a striking difference between the oral and intramuscular administration of MPA (Fig. 7). In the group of 10 patients on 100 mg MPA tablets twice daily, a plateau level of around 20 ng MPA per ml plasma was soon reached and maintained through the study. The monthly variations were mostly due to difficulties in obtaining the blood samples at constant and correct intervals after the last dose of MPA in this outpatient group. In both groups having MPA administered intramuscularly an accumulation of MPA was observed in the plasma levels. The two curves of the MPA levels ran parallel and throughout the study they correlate well to the doses given. From the first week intramuscular injections of 1000 mg MPA once

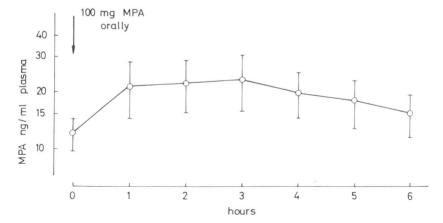

FIG. 5. Plasma concentrations of MPA after an oral dose of 100 mg MPA in a group of 8 patients treated for 12 weeks with 100 mg MPA twice daily. Mean ± SEM.

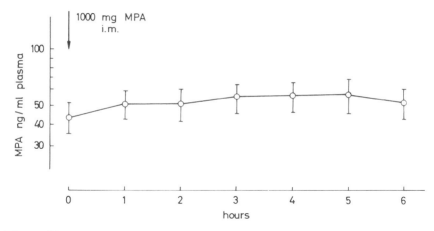

FIG. 6. Plasma concentrations of MPA after an i.m. dose of 1000 mg MPA in a group of 7 patients treated for 12 weeks with 1000 mg MPA once a week. Mean ± SEM.

a week gave higher blood levels than the oral administration of 100 mg MPA twice daily. The intramuscular doses of 1000 mg MPA every 2 weeks initially caused lower plasma levels but after 8–9 weeks the curve increased above the levels obtained in the tablet regimen.

In the group of 5 patients on 1000 mg MPA daily in oral administration a mean plasma level of 33 ng/ml was found after treatment for 7 days. After 14 and 21 days the plasma values were 27 and 24 ng/ml, respectively (Fig. 8). This decreasing plasma level is mostly due to very low values in one patient following high level on day 7.

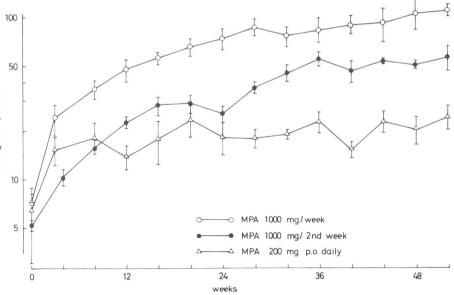

FIG. 7. Plasma concentrations of MPA in a long-term study of three different groups of 10 patients each on dosage schedules of 1000 mg MPA i.m. once a week, 1000 mg MPA i.m. once every 2 weeks, and 100 mg MPA twice daily in oral doses. Mean ± SEM.

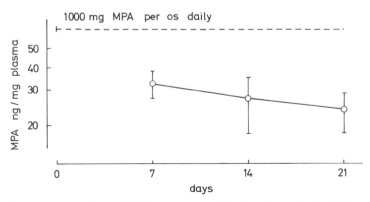

FIG. 8. Plasma concentrations of MPA in a group of 5 patients treated with 1000 mg MPA daily in oral administration. Mean ± SEM.

The daily intramuscular injections of 1000 mg MPA in 11 patients produced a mean plasma level increasing from 46 ng/ml day 7 to 91 ng/ml day 14 (Fig. 9). In a treatment schedule 4 patients were given loading daily doses of 1000 mg MPA intramuscularly for 14 days followed by a maintenance dose of 1000 mg MPA intramuscularly once weekly. From a level of 87 ng/ml at the end of the loading phase the mean plasma concentration decreases to 48 ng/ml after 2 weeks when two maintenance doses have been given (Fig. 10).

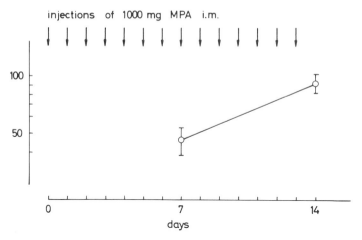

FIG. 9. Plasma concentrations of MPA in 11 patients treated with daily i.m. doses of 1000 mg MPA. Mean ± SEM.

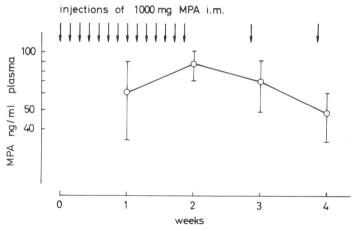

FIG. 10. Plasma concentrations of MPA in 4 patients treated with 1000 mg MPA in an i.m. administration daily for 14 days followed by the same dose once weekly. Mean ± SEM.

DISCUSSION

The plasma levels of MPA are directly related to the dose administered, whether orally or intramuscularly. There are considerable interindividual differences in all groups, but for the individual as for the mean plasma levels there seems to be a linear correlation between dose administered and the plasma values. A single oral dose of 100 or 200 mg produces higher peak levels than the values obtained after a single intramuscular injection of as much as 1000 mg MPA. From such an observation it might be concluded that by administration of equivalent weekly doses the oral route was better than the intramuscular. Such erroneous conclusions have in fact been drawn. Sall et al. (12) administered more than three times the amount of MPA in an oral dosage (150 mg daily) as in an intramuscular dosage (300 mg

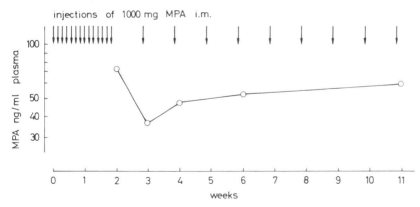

FIG. 11. Plasma concentrations of MPA in patient AH during i.m. administration of MPA 1000 mg daily for 2 weeks and then once a week.

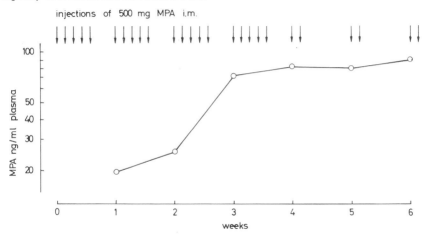

FIG. 12. Plasma concentrations of MPA in patient WV during i.m. administration of MPA 500 mg 5 days per week for 4 weeks and then twice a week.

weekly) and consequently reported significantly higher blood levels with the oral route. Laatikainen et al. (8) reported plasma values of the same order irrespective of whether the single MPA dose (100 mg) was given orally or intramuscularly. However, the depot effect of intramuscularly administered MPA is striking and is of the utmost importance in the long-term treatment of cancer patients (7).

Recently Maskens et al. (9) presented preliminary data from a study of MPA serum levels in different treatment schedules. Serum MPA was determined by gas liquid chromatography. In prolonged treatments (more than 8 weeks) serum MPA levels were found to be proportional to the administered dose, with markedly higher levels when using the intramuscular versus the oral route. These findings are consistent with the results of this study.

The cumulative effect with the intramuscular administration of MPA in our series showed considerable interindividual differences. In one patient a plasma level of

100 ng/ml was reached after 10 months with 1000 mg MPA given intramuscularly once weekly. In another patient values above this level were registered even after only 3 months on the same regimen.

It seems reasonable to assume that the steady increase in MPA concentration in plasma seen in the intramuscularly treated groups is attributable to the steady increase in new depot sites. MPA given intramuscularly has an excellent depot effect, with release of MPA from the injection site for up to 9 months (6).

The different patient groups in this study were not sufficiently numerous to allow conclusions to be drawn concerning adequate therapeutic plasma levels of MPA. This problem concerning therapeutic level and consequently the dosage problem in MPA treatment has not yet been properly elucidated in clinical studies. However, from clinical experience high MPA doses are more commonly used in the treatment of cancer. From this study it can be concluded that if it is necessary for the treatment effect to obtain a high plasma level of MPA (more than 50 ng/ml) the intramuscular administration of MPA is the method to be used. In further studies very high daily doses of MPA (2–5 g) administered by the oral route must be given if plasma levels in a range of 50–100 ng/ml should be obtained. In the treatment of cancer it is important to achieve effect as soon as possible. For that reason an MPA dosage schedule in which daily intramuscular loading doses are followed by weekly maintenance doses (Fig. 9) is preferable to a continuous treatment with equal amounts of MPA every week (Fig. 7). Two different models of such a MPA treatment are illustrated in Figs. 11 and 12.

REFERENCES

1. Anderson, D. C. (1965): *Am. J. Obstet. Gynecol.*, 113:195.
2. Babcock, Y. V., Gutselle, S., Heve, N. H., Hogg, Y. A., Stucky, Y. C., and Barnes, W. E. (1958): *J. Am. Chem. Soc.*, 80:2904.
3. Bonte, J. (1972): *Acta Obstet. Gynecol. Scand. Suppl.*, 19:21.
4. Cornette, J. C., Kirton, K. T., and Duncan, G. W. (1971): *J. Clin. Endocrinol. Metab.*, 33:459.
5. Decoster, J. M., Bonte, J., and Marco, A. (1977): *Gynecol. Oncol.*, 5:189.
6. Jeppsson, S., and Johansson, E. D. B. (1976): *Contraception*, 14:461.
7. Hesselius, I., and Johansson, E. D. B. (1981): *Acta Obstet. Gynecol. Scand. (in press)*.
8. Laatikainen, T., Nieminen, U., and Adlercreutz, H. (1979): *Acta Obstet. Gynecol. Scand.*, 58:95.
9. Maskens, A., Hap, B., Kazyreff, W. N., Gallewaert, W., Lion, G., and Van den Abbeele, K. (1980): *AACR Abstr.*, 661.
10. Ortiz, A., Hiroi, M., Stanczyk, F. Z., Goebelsman, U., and Mishell Jr., D. R. (1977): *J. Clin. Endocrinol. Metab.*, 44:32.
11. Sala, G., Camerino, B., and Cavallero, C. (1958): *Acta Endocrinol. (Kbh)*, 29:508.
12. Sall, S., Disaia, P., Morrow, P., Mortel, R., Prem, R., Thigpen, T., and Creasman, W. (1979): *Am. J. Obstet. Gynecol.*, 135:649.
13. Victor, A., and Johansson, E. D. B. (1976): *Contraception*, 14:319.

Role of Medroxyprogesterone in Endocrine-Related Tumors, Volume II, edited by L. Campio, G. Robustelli Della Cuna, and R. W. Taylor. Raven Press, New York © 1983.

High-Dose Medroxyprogesterone Acetate Therapy: Plasma Levels and Bioavailability-Response Correlation After Single and Multiple Dose Administration in Advanced Cancer Patients—Preliminary Results

F. Pannuti, *C. M. Camaggi, E. Strocchi, M. Giovannini, G. Iafelice, N. Canova, B. Costanti, and **G. Murari

*Oncology Division, M. Malpighi Hospital, 40138 Bologna, *Institute of Organic Chemistry, and **Institute of Pharmacology, University of Bologna, 40136 Bologna, Italy*

Medroxyprogesterone acetate (MPA, 6α-methyl-17α-hydroxyprogesterone acetate) is now widely used in advanced breast cancer therapy and has been found to be useful in the management of renal, prostatic, and endometrial tumors as well as in oncological pain control (1,6,9–11). *In vitro* studies show that MPA nearly inhibits the growth of the MCF 7 human breast cancer tumor cell line at 1×10^{-6} M (300 ng/ml) concentration, whereas it is ineffective at the lower 1×10^{-8} M level (2). These findings, together with the low toxicity of the drug, suggest that the goal of any therapeutical schedule must be to reach the maximum possible plasma drug level. Actually, it has already been proven, that the effectiveness of MPA treatment is greatly enhanced by using "high" daily doses ($\geqslant$ 500 mg/day) (8).

In common clinical practice, administration schedules still tend to be poorly defined. Intramuscular (i.m.) administration is probably more extensively used, although severe local intolerance often inhibits the prolonged use of the drug. Oral (o.p.) administration has been proven equally effective as i.m. treatment and devoid of its unnecessary side effects (7), but there is still no general agreement on the more effective dose schedule.

In order to throw some light on the still unresolved problems connected with the clinical use of high doses of MPA, our institute has initiated a multidisciplinary study on pharmacokinetic, metabolic, and clinical response following MPA treatments.

We report here some preliminary results concerning: (a) plasma MPA pharmacokinetics following i.m. and p.o. at single (500, 2000 mg) and multiple (500, 2000 mg/day) administration; (b) dose/bioavailability/clinical response correlations; (c) perspectives.

OUTLINE OF THE STUDY

Patients included in this study were hospital inpatients with histologically proven far-advanced cancer. All had received prior radiation therapy and/or chemo- or hormonotherapy, but oncological treatments were discontinued at least 1 month before the time of this study (generally because of lack of response). Throughout the experiment, commercially available MPA vials [FARLUTAL Depot (1000 mg/vials) Farmitalia] were used.

Oral treatments were performed using MPA suspension in fruit juice, while i.m. treatment was administered using either a single 500-mg injection (500 mg i.m. single and multiple treatments) or two subsequent 1000-mg injections (2000-mg single and multiple treatments). Blood samples were collected in the usual way and 1-ml plasma samples were analyzed for MPA levels with a gas-chromatographic procedure as described elsewhere (5).

Although the intrinsic cross-reactivity problems of the radioimmunoassay of MPA (12) can now be partially overcome by using a selective extraction technique, we preferred this chromatographic method because of the complete absence of interferences with MPA metabolites; its much better run to run coefficient of variation (8%), and its high linearity range (2–1000 ng/ml) (at the present time we have determined MPA concentration on time profiles in about 400 patients). Data processing was performed on a CDC Cyber 76 computer system using the SPSS package of programs for statistical analysis (3).

RESULTS

MPA Plasma Pharmacokinetic After Single Administration

Table 1 reports mean plasma levels of MPA following single dose administration, together with the 95% confidence interval [$\bar{X} \pm t (s \sqrt{N})$; s = standard deviation; t = Student's t for 0.025 probability and $N - 1$ degrees of freedom]; each value is the mean of determination in 10 cancer patients. In the single patients the time/concentration plot after p.o. administration shows some discontinuities, but mean curves are reasonably smooth and can be easily interpolated by a triexponential function (13):

$$(C) = A \cdot \exp (\alpha t) + B \cdot \exp (\beta t) + C \cdot \exp (\gamma t)$$

The parameters obtained by the best-fit procedure (5) are reported in Table 2. After p.o. administration, mean plasma levels rapidly increased, reaching a peak in about 2 hr (Fig. 1).

Following this peak was biexponential decay characterized by an initial half-life ($t\frac{1}{2}$) of about 2 hr and a terminal phase of about 35 hr. However, while the determination of initial half-life is sufficiently accurate, the second one probably suffers from the lower accuracy of this analytical method at plasma levels below that of about 2 ng/ml.

TABLE 1. *Mean plasma levels (ng/ml) after single-dose o.p. and i.m. administration (10 advanced cancer patients/group)*

Time (hr)	500 mg p.o.		2000 mg p.o.		500 mg i.m.		2000 mg i.m.	
	X	C.I.	X	C.I.	X	C.I.	X	C.I.
0	0.0		0.0		0.0		0.0	
1	6.7	(2.7–10.7)	18.1	(6.3–29.8)	4.5	(1.7–7.3)	8.6	(0.0–18.4)
2	9.9	(4.6–15.1)	29.9	(9.6–50.3)	4.0	(1.4–6.6)	8.9	(1.9–15.9)
4	9.4	(3.5–15.3)	24.6-	(12.2–36.9)	3.9	(1.7–6.2)	9.3	(4.9–13.6)
6	5.9	(3.4–8.4)	15.7	(7.1–24.3)	3.6	(2.0–5.3)	6.7	(3.0–10.3)
8	3.0	(1.3–4.7)	10.9	(4.0–17.8)	4.1	(2.9–5.9)	7.7	(4.6–10.8)
26	2.3	(1.2–3.4)	4.2	(1.4–6.9)	4.2	(1.7–6.4)	9.3	(4.4–14.1)
50	1.6	(1.0–2.3)	0.9	(0.0–2.2)	2.9	(1.6–4.4)	10.0	(5.4–14.6)
74	1.2	(0.4–2.0)	1.3	(0.2–2.4)	3.6	(0.2–6.9)	9.9	(4.5–15.2)
98	1.2	(0.3–2.2)	1.0	(0.0–2.2)	3.5	(1.6–5.5)	11.5	(1.7–21.4)
164	0.9	(0.2–1.7)	1.0	(0.1–2.0)	3.9	(2.3–5.4)	11.1	(6.2–16.2)

X = average value; p.o. = oral route; C.I. = 95% confidence interval; i.m. = intramuscular route.

TABLE 2. *Interpolation of absorption/decay after oral administration*

Parameters	500 mg	1000 mg	2000 mg
A	− 78.04	− 44.44	− 499.01
B	76.22	42.46	429.35
C	1.6	2.03	5.95
α	− 0.513	− 0.977	− 0.481
$t \frac{1}{2} \alpha$	1.35	0.71	1.44
β	− 0.374	− 0.445	− 0.420
$t \frac{1}{2} \beta$	1.85	1.52	1.65
γ	a	a	− 0.020
γ	a	a	35.65
M.S.E.	0.28	0.04	1.49

M.S.E. = mean square error.
a: Because of the low accuracy of the analytical method below 2 ng/ml, these data are scarcely significant.

The simplest pharmacokinetic model which correctly explained the observed plasma decay is a two-compartment open model. The first decay phase can be attributed to the distribution in peripheral tissues, and is obscured by the prolonged absorption phase after i.m. administration (Fig. 1).

It is of particular interest to note the different behavior of the MPA plasma levels after p.o. and i.m. administration. Peak levels are much higher after p.o. treatment, but a much better long-term bioavailability is obtained after i.m. administration, due to the prolonged absorption phase.

Areas under the time/concentration curves (AUC) are reported in Table 3. Aside from the high interindividual variance, the relationship between administered dose and AUC (and therefore the bioavailability of the drug) is statistically significant.

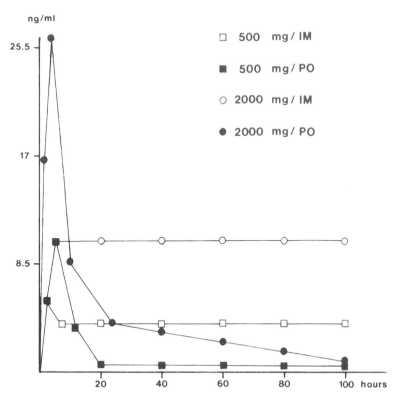

FIG. 1. Mean plasma MPA levels following single o.p. or i.m. administration.

TABLE 3. *Area under absorption/decay curve [(ng/hr/ml⁻¹)10⁻³]:*
Single administration (o.p. and i.m. route)

500 mg p.o.		2000 mg p.o.		500 mg i.m.		2000 mg i.m.	
BG	0.126	AA	0.454	BL	0.404	GG	0.668
BI	0.227	CG	0.894	BS	0.358	GM	3.960
MC	0.291	LF	0.382	FR	0.398	GO	1.096
ME	0.064	MC	0.587	MI	0.173	MA	2.702
CA	0.256	SA	0.400	RA	0.669	MC	1.435
MA	0.336	TR	0.141	RM	0.250	RM	1.248
PE	0.276	ML	0.985	MF	0.470	SC	0.536
CZ	0.409	TR	0.358	ZO	1.423	BM	1.295
PG	0.251	ZD	0.296	ME	0.422	MA	0.638
DE	0.309	CL	0.125	BC	0.464	BM	1.451
Mean value	0.255		0.442		0.503		1.503
± SE	±0.005		±0.096		±0.110		±0.335

SE = standard error; p.o = oral route; i.m. = intramuscular route.

MPA Plasma Levels and Bioavailability After Multiple Administration

MPA plasma levels after multiple administration (500 and 2000 mg/day p.o. or i.m. for 30 days; 5 cancer patients in each group) are reported in Table 4 and Fig. 2.

The depot effect observed after single i.m. treatment is particularly evident here. In the first 4 days of the therapy, higher plasma levels are present after o.p. administration. Yet after this initial period, i.m. treatment shows a relatively higher bioavailability. After the last dose, MPA plasma levels after p.o. administration decay with a half-life of about 2 days and after i.m. treatment remain stable. Both plasma levels and AUC (Table 5) are dose-dependent. Furthermore, it is important to note that p.o. treatment requires a much higher daily dose than the i.m. route to reach the equivalent bioavailability.

MPA Bioavailability and Clinical Response

The wide intersubject spread observed in MPA plasma levels and following both single and multiple administration, indicates that any statistical analysis of dose/response relationships will very likely be affected by an additional discriminant factor, i.e., the actual percentage of absorbed drug. We therefore tried to directly correlate the clinical response to MPA therapy with the effective drug bioavailability—rather than with the administered dose—in the single patients (as measured by AUC values and MPA plasma levels).

Two clinical parameters have been taken in account at this stage of our work: objective response (determined according to UICC standards) in a group of 27 patients with advanced hormono-sensitive tumors and pain response in a group of 31 patients. MPA plasma levels were determined during the treatment, and areas under the AUC calculated in the 0–37-day interval.

Figure 3 reports mean MPA plasma levels during a typical 30-day treatment, by objective response category. Comparison of this graph with the data reported in

TABLE 4. *Mean plasma levels (ng/ml) after multiple doses (o.p. and i.m. administration; 5 advanced cancer patients/group)*

Time (days)	500 mg/day p.o. $\overline{X}$	C.I.	2000 mg/day p.o. $\overline{X}$	C.I.	500 mg/day i.m. $\overline{X}$	C.I.	2000 mg/day i.m. $\overline{X}$	C.I.
4	19.7	(0.0–39.4)	29.6	(13.6–45.6)	9.7	(7.1–12.2)	36.3	(26.1–46.5)
8	18.5	(0.0–39.9)	69.6	(17.3–121.8)	23.8	(0.0–58.9)	99.8	(48.0–151.6)
12	15.5	(0.0–41.7)	75.2	(16.9–133.5)	44.4	(0.0–97.8)	122.0	(36.0–208.0)
15	30.1	(0.0–61.2)	77.2	(10.4–144.0)	47.2	(6.0–88.4)	150.8	(61.2–240.4)
21	16.0	(3.6–28.4)	86.4	(8.1–164.7)	43.2	(15.2–71.1)	200.9	(88.8–312.1)
28	14.0	(0.5–27.5)	63.2	(11.8–114.6)	53.6	(10.8–96.4)	251.8	(119.9–383.7)
30	7.9	(6.9–9.7)	67.2	(24.1–110.3)	64.0	(33.1–94.9)	303.7	(131.5–475.9)
31	4.2	(2.7–5.7)	30.1	(25.7–34.4)	58.1	(28.0–88.1)	258.6	(156.8–360.4)
33	3.0	(0.0–7.0)	22.2	(8.0–36.5)	44.5	(20.3–68.7)	290.6	(183.1–398.1)
35	1.9	(0.0–5.0)	11.4	(3.4–19.4)	43.7	(18.0–69.4)	246.3	(119.3–375.3)
37	0.0	(0.0–0.0)	4.3	(1.2–77.4)	49.6	(14.5–84.6)	286.6	(146.1–427.0)

$\overline{X}$ = mean value; p.o. = oral route; C.I. = 95% confidence interval; i.m. = intramuscular route.

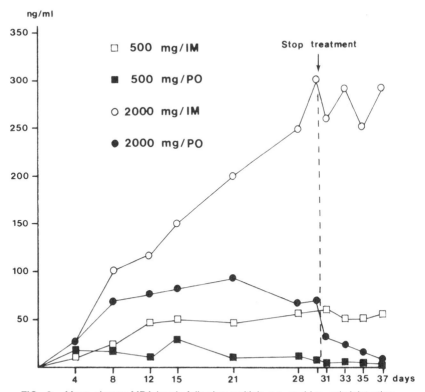

FIG. 2. Mean plasma MPA levels following multiple o.p. and i.m. administration.

TABLE 5. *Area under absorption/decay curve: Multiple-dose administration*
(o.p. and i.m. route)

500 mg p.o.		2000 mg p.o.		500 mg i.m.		2000 mg i.m.	
SR	5.11	GG	42.23	CC	67.88	RG	131.89
GAM	6.02	CD	91.14	BE	19.56	FE	229.33
BM	24.87	CI	16.24	RA	25.96	FI	158.61
ME	16.84	MF	43.77	SI	22.23	LG	103.29
SM	11.31	PS	57.34	GB	36.28	BM	110.52
Mean value	12.83		50.14		34.38		146.73
± SE	±3.67		±12.22		±8.84		±22.78

AUC = (ng/hr/ml^{-1}) × 10^{-3}; p.o. = oral route; SE = standard error; i.m. = intramuscular route.

Table 4 and Fig. 2, indicates that the mean levels observed in responders can only be reached by using very high daily doses.

Tables 6 and 7 report the clinical responses to the MPA therapy correlated with the AUC values, indication of the effective bioavailability of the drug in the single patients. For AUC values of less than 50 × 10^{-3}, MPA treatments seem to be

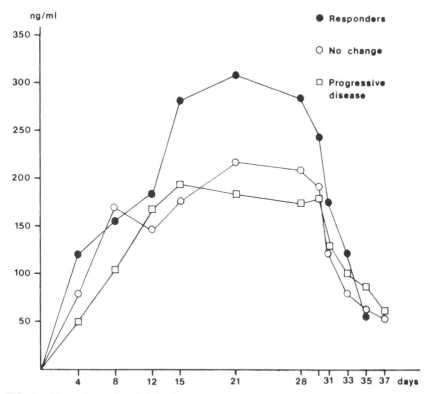

FIG. 3. Mean plasma levels following treatment with MPA by objective response category.

TABLE 6. *Treatment of far-advanced cancer patients with multiple high doses of MPA: Comparison of objective response with bioavailability*

Area (ng/hr/ml⁻¹) × 10⁻³	R	NC	P
<200	3/27 (11%)	3/27 (11%)	2/27 (7%)
101–200	0/27 (—)	6/27 (22%)	2/27 (7%)
51–100	2/27 (7%)	2/27 (7%)	0/27 (—)
<50	0/27 (—)	3/27 (11%)	4/27 (15%)
Total	5/27 (18.5%)	14/27 (52%)	8/27 (29.5%)
$\chi^2 = 11.63$		$p < 0.07$	

R = partial + minimal remission; NC = no change; P = progression.

scarcely effective both in pain control and antiblastic action. It is to be noted that low AUC values, and therefore unfavorable clinical responses, were obtained in some cases after administration of very high MPA dosages (in one case, for instance, patient BC received a treatment of 3000 mg/p.o./daily and AUC was only 12×10^{-3}).

TABLE 7. *Patients with advanced cancer. Treatment with multiple high doses of MPA: Comparison of pain response with bioavailability*

Area $(ng/hr/ml^{-1}) \times 10^{-3}$	R	NC	P
>200	4/31(13%)	1/31(3%)	1/31(3%)
101–200	4/31(13%)	4/31(13%)	1/31(3%)
51–100	3/31(10%)	3/31(10%)	1/31(3%)
<50	1/31(3%)	5/31(16%)	3/31(10%)
Pearson's $R = -0.346$		$p < 0.03$	

R = pain relief; P = progression; NC = no change.

Globally, there is an indication that higher MPA bioavailability improves both pain and objective responses. Notwithstanding the limited number of data still available, statistical analysis of these contingency tables actually confirms that this trend is significant. To improve clinical use, further studies have been carried out to test whether patients, affected by the most common tumors and metastases, show some systemic MPA absorption pattern.

In particular, discriminant analysis (3) was applied to a group of 101 patients receiving single doses of MPA, and grouped according to a previously reported classification (4) based on the site and number of metastases. No statistically significant differences were observed, except for a group of 11 patients with liver metastases, who showed higher MPA plasma levels. These results were not surprising, since liver takes part in MPA metabolism, and substantial quantities of MPA were found in bile of a patient 2 hr after the administration of a single 2000 mg/p.o. dose.

PERSPECTIVE

It looks promising, on the basis of the results reported above, to follow dosage regimens that guarantee high MPA bioavailability, which can be achieved by using very high MPA dosages or checking MPA plasma levels in the single patients, and then adjusting the therapy according to the analytical data. We are currently exploring alternative methods to find the optimization of MPA treatment schedules, such as tests on new dosage forms or alternative modes of administration, and which give better absorption efficiencies.

After simultaneous administration of 1000 mg i.m., we observed mean plasma profiles, that were exactly the superimposition of the two absorption/decay curves, obtained after administration of the single dose i.m. or p.o.

The simultaneous administration of MPA by i.m. and p.o. route may be effective in overcoming the drawbacks of both routes—i.e., the local intolerance sometimes observed in high dose i.m. treatment and the low percentage of absorbed drug, typical of the p.o. administration. Intramuscular doses can guarantee long-term MPA plasma levels with low incidence of side effects, while the simultaneous administration of higher daily p.o. doses will increase MPA plasma levels into therapeutic range.

CONCLUSION

This pharmacokinetic study of MPA has potential clinical application: delineation of drug concentration consistent with clinical response and determination of an appropriate dose schedule to rapidly achieve drug levels consistent with response. As shown from the results concerning both single and multiple administration, MPA is absorbed by oral route and can be safely given per os in common clinical practice to patients; it must be clearly pointed out that the use of very high MPA doses per os finds its rationale on the low absorption efficiency observed for the currently available drug preparations.

As shown above, in order to reach consistently steady-state plasma levels of 100 ng/ml (i.e., concentration of about 2.5×10^{-7} M) it is mandatory to use daily doses of at least 2000 mg, when for other water-soluble related drugs—as, for instance, tamoxifen—the same level is easily reached with 20 mg/day. With such high dosages involved, the fact of the "not-absorbed" drug becomes highly relevant; we are currently studying in detail the MPA tissue distribution and metabolism. Comparison of response by bioavailability or plasma levels indicate that—if the trend observed in our preliminary study is confirmed—some accepted treatment schedules may in some cases give subtherapeutic MPA levels.

REFERENCES

1. Concolino, G., Marocchi, A., Conti, C., Tenaglia, R., Di Silverio, F., and Bracci, U. (1978): *Cancer Res.*, 38:4340.
2. Di Marco, A. (1980): *Role of Medroxyprogesterone in Endocrine-Related Tumors*, edited by S. Iacobelli and A. Di Marco, pp. 1–20. Raven Press, New York.
3. Nie, N. H., Hull, C. H., Jenkins, J. G., Steinbrenner, K., and Bent, D. H. (1980): *SPSS Statistical Package for the Social Sciences*, 2nd ed. McGraw Hill, New York.
4. Pannuti, F. (1977): Il protocollo terapeutico e i codici di caratterizzazione e di valutazione in clinica oncologica, edited by F. Pannuti. Editrice Universitaria Bolognese, Bologna.
5. Pannuti, F., Cammagi, C. M., Strocchi, E., Giovannini, M., Di Marco, A. R., and Costanti, B. (1981): *Cancer Treat Rep. (in press)*.
6. Pannuti, F., Camaggi, C. M., Strocchi, E., Giovannini, M., Lippi, A., and Canova, N. (1981): *Cancer Treat. Rep. (in press)*.
7. Pannuti, F., Martoni, A., Di Marco, A. R., Piana, E., et al. (1979): *Europ. J. Cancer*, 15:593–601.
8. Pannuti, F., Martoni, A., Fruet, F., Strocchi, E., and Di Marco, A. R. (1979): *Breast Cancer Experimental and Clinical Aspects*, edited by H. T. Mouridsen and T. Palshof, pp. 93–98. Pergamon Press, London.
9. Pannuti, F., Martoni, A., Lenaz, G. R., Piana, E., and Nanni, P. (1978): *Cancer Treat. Rep.*, 62:499–504.
10. Pannuti, F., Martoni, A., Rossi, A. P., and Piana, E. (1979): *Advances in Pain Research and Therapy*, Vol. 2, edited by Y. Y. Bonica and V. Ventafridda, pp. 145–165. Raven Press, New York.
11. Pannuti, F., Rossi, A. P., and Piana, E. (1977): *IRCS*, 5:375.
12. Rendina, G. M., and Donadio, C. (1975): *Min. Gin.*, 27:1–5.
13. Salimtschik, M., Mouridsen, H. T., Loeber, J., and Johansson, E. (1980): *Cancer Chemother. Pharmacol.*, 4:267–269.
14. Wagner, J. G. (1975): *Fundamentals of Clinical Pharmacokinetics*, 3rd ed. Drug Intelligence Publication, Hamilton, New York.

Role of Medroxyprogesterone in Endocrine-Related Tumors, Volume II, edited by L. Campio, G. Robustelli Della Cuna, and R. W. Taylor. Raven Press, New York © 1983.

Medroxyprogesterone Acetate and Tamoxifen: Two Different Drugs in Alternate or Sequential Modality Treatment

A. Pellegrini, B. Massidda, V. Mascia, and M. T. Ionta

Institute of Clinical Oncology, Cagliari Medical School and General Cancer Hospital, 09100 Cagliari, Italy

Clinical results and the slow but continuous progress in endocrine pathophysiology of hormone-related tumors allow some considerations about their actual treatment strategy, mainly in regard to advanced breast cancer. Oophorectomy, antiestrogens, high-dose progestins, and aminogluthetimide represent the actual main hormonal manipulations: the median response rate is about 30% with a median response duration of about 12 months. The receptors monitor treatment almost doubles the response rate without a really significant increase of the response duration; at the same time we have very little evidence of overall survival prolongation.

Chemotherapy also reached a stable response rate around 50% and chemo-hormonotherapy, introduced as a more aggressive combined modality treatment based on the rationale of different sensitive cell populations to chemo- or hormonotherapy alone, is still in an experimental phase without any definite evidence of its superiority in regard to overall survival, quality of life, better combinations, sequences, and schedules.

Therefore an apparent "plateau" of clinical results has been reached in advanced breast cancer treatment but, at the same time, the endocrine pathophysiology of breast, endometrial, and prostatic tumors underwent some quite impressive progress (24).

Experimental and clinical investigations into hormone receptors and the pathogenic role played by hormones in breast cancer have provided a deeper insight into the involved hormonal relations, specific and nonspecific hormone-receptor modulation for individual hormones, hormone binding, receptor-hormone complex translocation to and processing within the nucleus, and the role played by each hormone in controlling tumor growth. In short, on the basis of present knowledge, which however is not at all final, we can say that for each hormone-related tumor a specific endocrine-modulating complex exists that controls tumor growth and influences tumor response to treatment. For instance, unopposed estrogens, along with an-

45

drogens and prolactin, are now considered as the main messengers stimulating breast and endometrial cancer growth. Next to these hormones, also known as "major" hormones on account of their important pathogenic role, a number of "minor" hormones, such as insulin, prostaglandins, and gonadotropin are supposed to be also involved.

In prostatic carcinoma such a stimulating role is apparently played by androgens, with the contribution of prolactin and luteinizing hormone; protective functions seem to be performed by progestins.

Although still relatively vague, the above observations have already raised several biological and physiopathologic problems (Fig. 1), leading investigators to question some aspects of the therapeutic strategy of these tumors. For instance, a number of therapeutical responses that can neither be related to the individual's receptor concentration nor be accounted for by our present knowledge of endocrine mechanism, have led investigators (not without a good deal of uncertainty) to hold different opinions as to dosage levels and treatment schedules. Moreover, while physiological hormone levels allow any hormone to act as a messenger only by interacting with its specific receptor, it seems that high-dose hormones may also act through specific receptors for other hormones. This might account for the Huggins' phenomenon whereby a tumor responds both to deprivation or high doses of the same hormone. At the same time, this is a complication in therapeutic strategy design for individual cases, and makes the selection of effective drug combinations and dosages a rather empirical process. In addition, and most important because of the side effects caused by certain therapeutic regimens, standard hormone levels for additive endocrine therapy usually exceed physiological hormone levels by far, and consequently may produce a direct cytotoxic effect on both normal and tumor cells in addition to an indeterminable amount of real endocrine activity. One can then suspect (but not state) that lower doses and/or different sequences might improve therapeutic results, thus lowering the side effects. Finally, an important problem of the combined chemohormonal treatment is the resultant in cellular kinetics induced by the hormonal component in regard to the phase-specificity of

---

1. Positive or negative receptor patients respectively unresponding or responding to hormonal treatment

2. False receptor negativity depending on temporary endocrine conditions of the patients

3. A positive receptor doesn't mean an active receptor

4. Some hormonal doses are completely far from the endocrine-related tumors pathophysiology with a dose/side effects relationship

5. Hormone in high doses may also act through not specific receptors (Pg versus glucocorticoids or DHT receptors, DHT versus E_2 receptors)

6. Response increased rate of positive receptor patients to hormonal manipulation is not paralleled by significantly increased response duration

---

FIG. 1. Hormono-related tumors: Open Problems.

chemotherapy itself. The overall cytocidal effect might be altered by reduced or inhibited proliferation of hormone-dependent cells. Therefore, doubts remain as to which drug combinations are the best, and which sequences and doses are the most useful and optimum, especially for the single hormone included in each combination.

That is why results obtained so far and physiopathologic problems are consistently intricate and cause uncertainty and conflicting opinions; on the other hand the literature, only partly univocal, hardly provides any guidance.

This implies not only continuous uncertainty as to which treatment program can give the best prognostic result in terms of quality and quantity, but also differences in opinions on drug use. Today, the most frequently adopted treatments are anti-estrogen and progestin therapy; however, it is not hard for a clinical oncologist to read several conflicting papers about the primary role of one drug over the other, conceptual differences on chemohormonal combinations and, occasionally also reports showing incomplete understanding by their authors of the pharmacological properties of the compounds being compared.

Of course, better understanding of some therapeutic regimens and their best results can only be obtained through controlled studies in large samples and for sufficiently long periods of time. However, despite our present limited information and the reservation that may be made as to its future development, we feel it is possible and useful to outline a therapeutic strategy based on and reflecting a critical interpretation of the endocrine physiopathology in hormone-related tumors and the specific characteristics of the applied hormones—this being particularly important for antiestrogens and progestins—as well as of the modality for their administration (i.e., administered alone, in an alternate or sequential modality, or in combination with chemotherapeutic agents) (Fig. 2).

ANTIESTROGENS AND PROGESTINS

During the past few years, several antiestrogens were tested for efficacy especially in breast cancer. Tamoxifen (TAM), nafoxidine, and clomiphene are said to possess

1. DEEPER KNOWLEDGE OF MECHANISM OF ACTION OF THE COMMONLY APPLIED HORMONES AND ANTI-HORMONES

2. TREATMENT SCHEDULES OUTLINED UNDER IMPROVED CONNECTIONS WITH THE SPECIFIC TUMOR PHYSIOPATHOLOGY

3. POSSIBILITY TO APPLY NON-CROSS RESISTANT SCHEDULES IN SEQUENTIAL OR ALTERNATE MODALITY.

4. PILOT STUDIES WITH DIFFERENT HORMONAL COMBINATIONS AND DOSES BASED ON THE RATIONALE OF SINGLE TUMOR ENDOCRINE PHYSIOPATHOLOGY.

5. DEEP CONSIDERATION TO QUALITY AND DURATION OF THE OVERALL SURVIVAL.

FIG. 2. Hormono-related tumors treatment strategy: Operational bases.

identical spectra of activity and similar efficacy on neoplastic cells. However, only TAM is used on a large clinical scale and this must largely be ascribed to its low incidence of untoward effects. Despite the fact that clinical results are still changing and its pharmacological properties are still being studied, several exhaustive review and clinical papers have already been published (8–27).

Progestins, in particular megestrol, norethisterone, and medroxyprogesterone acetate (MPA) have been tested for many years, above all in mammary and endometrial carcinomas. Their effectiveness is very similar, and their response rates compare quite favorably to one another. Many years ago, MPA was tested in clinical studies of mammary carcinoma by the so-called low doses (100–200 mg/day); the reported impression was that progestins were not an important therapeutic weapon, and they were abandoned almost completely. However, during the past few years, this progestational agent was tested again at much higher dosages (500–1500 mg/day) and outstanding results were reported in the literature (6–12).

The rationale underlying the therapeutic applications of both drugs is to be found in the endocrine physiopathologic processes involved in human breast cancer, and in the effects these drugs produce on the specific hormone modulating system of this type of cancer. Moreover, MPA, being a progestational agent, is also effective in advanced endometrial and prostatic cancer. TAM, an antiestrogen, is not likely to be applied in prostatic carcinoma, but can be effective—at least under some defined criteria—in endometrial carcinoma.

If we consider breast cancer only, we can say that both TAM and MPA, and their specific effects, are not mutually exclusive from the point of view of therapeutic strategy. In fact, they can be used alternatively as the primary treatment within different therapeutic regimens for breast cancer therapy, depending on the patient's clinical and biochemical data. In pilot trials, and within the limits allowed by some of their pharmacological properties, both drugs might also be effectively included in alternate, sequential hormone regimens, closely reflecting some biological aspects of endometrial and mammary carcinoma to be discussed later (1,23).

DRUG PROPERTIES AND MECHANISMS OF ACTION

TAM is a nonsteroidal antiestrogen with a partial estrogen-agonistic activity. Its mechanism of action has not yet been completely elucidated, and the only confirmed property of the drug is its ability to compete for estradiol binding sites.

As estrogen is one of the "major" hormones involved in the specific endocrine modulation system of breast cancer, and has a stimulating effect on tumor growth (along with prolactin and androgens and without adequate progestational protection), the above-mentioned competition by antiestrogen for estrogen receptors represents the rationale underlying the clinical application of TAM (8,22).

An interesting assumption can be made, which is that TAM can induce chemical ovariectomy, on the basis of a few experimental data demonstrating its efficacy in lowering the levels of circulating estrogens. Consequently, in view of the relationship between estrogen and prolactin, the above effect is also supposed to reduce estrogen stimulation of the prolactin-producing cells; as a result of these effects, TAM seems to inhibit hormone stimulation of tumor growth (13–22). In practice, the mean value of prolactin fall is smaller than the one observed in ovariectomized animals, and this might be related to the amount of estrogen-like activity produced by certain dosage levels of TAM. On the other hand, in a group of premenopausal women treated with TAM, estrogen concentrations were high also in disease remission. This is a finding that can hardly be explained because of the low number of controlled studies of hormone level changes during antiestrogenic therapy; one can also speculate on increased gonadotropin levels in non-ovariectomized women, as a response could be obtained following ovariectomy in patients who did not respond any more to TAM (8). That is why ovariectomy seems to be a rational measure to couple with antiestrogen treatment in premenopausal women with metastasized tumor; as a matter of fact the endocrine rebound that might be stimulated in the ovaries by gonadotropin, and the resulting high levels of estrogen and probably prolactin, should be considered as negative events in the endocrine control system of tumor growth.

Like estradiol, TAM can translocate receptor complexes to nuclear sites, but it does not stimulate the synthesis of DNA-dependent RNA polymerase. The translocation process has been controversial, but now it is held that it depends upon dosage levels used by individual investigators (8).

It is interesting to note that estradiol increases the amount of DNA in endometrial cells and their mitotic index, thus causing the endometrium to become really hyperplastic, whereas TAM increases only cell volume, and does not induce cell mitosis (8). As to one of the messenger roles played by estrogen, it specifically consists in "priming" progesterone receptors in the target tissue.

It has been demonstrated that TAM and one of its active metabolites can stimulate the replenishment of the cytoplasmic progesterone receptors on a dose-related basis: medium doses appear to produce a larger amount of stimulation, whereas high, clearly antiestrogenic doses, depress progesterone receptor synthesis. After high TAM doses, cell growth is inhibited, and cell death may follow (8–10).

Stimulation of cytoplasmic progesterone receptors in hormone-related cells would combine its effect with the direct antiestrogenic action of TAM in a favorable way. Probably, this combined effect restores the cell's ability to respond to endogenous or exogenous progestin, which is an essential condition necessary to control tumor growth effectively and to modify the patient's hormonal environment in such a way as to impair the continued growth of an estrogen-dependent tumor. It is worthwhile stressing that a direct correlation exists between the cytoplasmic estrogen receptor content in the target tissue (i.e., the tumor) and tumor regression as induced by antiestrogens. Practically, no evidence is available that any endocrine- or hormone-antagonizing treatment can completely eradicate cancer because tumors contain cells with a varying degree of hormone-dependence, including total independence from hormones for their own growth. This observation, as well as complementary ones, have led investigators to view combination chemotherapy plus antiestrogen and progestational agents as a more aggressive approach to cancer therapy, and this is demonstrated by the number of experimental and clinical studies of its efficacy.

Recently, it was also assumed that TAM may inhibit prostaglandin-synthetase. In mammary carcinoma with bone metastases, a high amount of osteolysis occurs. Several factors, including prostaglandin-like material produced by the carcinoma itself, may be held responsible for that. In particular, the prostaglandin-like material is supposed to stimulate osteoclastic activity, thus leading to calcium mobilization and bone resorption, as demonstrated by clinical evidence and laboratory data (26–28).

By its assumed inhibiting effect on prostaglandin-synthetase, TAM would control cancer-induced bone resorption. Obviously, this is just a working hypothesis based on mostly *in vitro* results. However, this hypothesis is a suggestive concept in agreement with clinical results obtained with TAM in breast cancer patients with skeletal metastases. This is another example of the way TAM apparently interferes with an important process in the specific endocrine control system of this type of tumor. By this it should not be inferred that no other drug mechanism of action is involved; in particular, mention must be made here of TAM's direct cytotoxic effect on metastatic cells, and—probably—a certain amount of estrogen-like effect produced by it on the mechanisms regulating the calcium-phosphate balance and the osteolysis-osteosynthesis mechanisms.

Another hypothesis has been put forth recently on the basis of studies on tumor growth and neoangiogenic factors that enable the tumor to control its own environment in a way that promotes the growth itself. It was assumed that a prostaglandin may be invoved in the neoangiogenic processes, and that by inhibiting its effect, angiogenesis might be reduced, and tumor growth might also be impaired or reduced (7). Therefore it may be hypothesized that on account of its prostaglandin-synthetase inhibiting activity, TAM is likely to affect the cell environment at the metastasized bone level. A similar mechanism might partially be responsible for the pain-relieving effect reported after TAM treatment by patients with skeletal metastases.

In short (Figs. 3–5) TAM mainly possesses an antiestrogenic effect and competes for cytoplasmic estrogen binding sites; moreover, at certain dosage levels, it shows a relative amount of estrogen-like activity. It is also speculated that it may lower circulating prolactin levels through inhibition of estrogen stimulation of hypophyseal prolactin-producing cells. It also antagonizes prostaglandin, probably via prostaglandin-synthetase inhibition, and this might account for the favorable effect produced by it on bone resorption when skeletal metastases are present. Lastly, as a result of its estrogen-like effect (at least at certain dosage levels), TAM can stimulate the replenishment of the cytoplasmic progesterone receptors thereby rendering sequential treatment with progestational agents possible for mammary and endometrial carcinoma.

MPA, a synthetic steroidal derivative of progesterone, posseses specific progestational effect and antiestrogenic, antiandrogenic, and antigonadotropinic activity; however its mechanisms of action have not yet been completely elucidated (Figs. 6–7). MPA acts through its interaction with specific progestin receptors, and inhibits

1. ESTROGEN BINDING COMPETITIVE INHIBITION AT RECEPTORS LEVEL

2. POSSIBLE CHEMICAL OOPHORECTOMY(LOWERED CIRCULATING ESTROGEN)

3. PROSTAGLANDINS (PGE_2-PGF_2)-SYNTHETASE INHIBITION.

4. POSSIBLE TUMOR ANGIOGENIC FACTOR(S) BLOCKADE THROUGH PROS-
   TAGLANDINS INHIBITION.

5. DOSE-DEPENDENT ESTROGEN-AGONISTIC ACTIVITY.

6. REDUCTION OF TARGET CELL'S PROLACTIN RECEPTORS CONTENT(animal).

FIG. 3. Tamoxifen: Mechanisms of action.

1. REDUCTION OR INHIBITION OF ESTROGEN-STIMULATED PROLACTIN RE-
   LEASE.

2. INTERFERENCE ON METASTATIC OSTEOLYTIC PROCESSES THROUGH PROS-
   TAGLANDINS.

3. INTERFERENCE ON BONE PAIN POSSIBLY THROUGH PROSTAGLANDINS.

4. POSSIBLE DIRECT ACTIVITY ON TUMOR GROWTH THROUGH NEO-ANGIOGE-
   NIC FACTOR(S).

5. DOSE-DEPENDENT "PRIMING" ACTIVITY FOR PROGESTERONE RECEPTORS.

6. STILL DEBATED ACTIVITY ON GONADOTROPINS CIRCULATING LEVELS.

FIG. 4. Tamoxifen: General activity.

TAMOXIFEN INTERFERES ON BREAST CANCER SPECIFIC "ENDOCRINE MODULATING COMPLEX"
ESSENTIALLY THROUGH :

1. REDUCTION OR INHIBITION OF ESTROGEN, PROLACTIN AND PROSTAGLANDINS
   ACTIVITIES.

2. DOSE-RELATED CELL "PRIMING" OF PROGESTERONE RECEPTORS.

3. POSSIBLE INHIBITION OF TUMOR GROWTH FACILITATING NEO ANGIOGENIC
   FACTOR(S).

FIG. 5. Tamoxifen: Role in breast cancer treatment.

cancer cell growth through direct action on tumor tissue, that is, it modifies the
specific tumor endocrine control system, and the patient's hormonal environment.
Present medium-high doses of MPA clearly produce a direct cytotoxic effect, which
is very likely to result (but partially) from MPA interaction with progesterone
receptors. In fact, as said above, MPA may interfere with hydrocortisone and

1. CIRCULATING ANDROGENS DECREASE

2. DECREASED ANDROGENS BINDING TO TeBG

3. LIVER INDUCTION OF A-RING-TESTOSTERONE REDUCTASE (IN-
   CREASED METABOLISM)

4. REDUCED CONVERSION FROM ANDROGENS TO ESTROGENS

5. ANDROGENS RECEPTORS COMPETITION (?)

6. FSH-LH SECRETION BLOCKADE

7. COMPETITION WITH ESTROGENS AT RECEPTOR LEVEL (DECREA-
   SING EFFECT ?)

8. ACCELERATION OF ESTROGENS ENZYMATIC CATABOLISM (E_2 -
   DEHYDROGENASE)

9. DIRECT CYTOTOXIC ACTION (DOSE RELATED)

10. ESTROGEN-PROGESTINS INTERACTION AND SYNERGISM AT RECEP-
    TOR LEVELS (?)

FIG. 6.   Progestational steroids: Possible mechanisms of action.

MEDROXYPROGESTERONE INTERFERES ON BREAST CANCER SPECIFIC "ENDOCRINE MODULATING
COMPLEX" ESSENTIALLY THROUGH :

1. MODIFICATION OF ANDROGENIC ENVIRONMENT AND REDUCED ANDROGEN-ESTROGEN
   CONVERSION.

2. REDUCED TARGET CELL EXPOSITION TO ACTIVE ESTROGENS.

3. DECREASED ESTROGEN AND PROLACTIN RECEPTORS. REPLENISHMENT.

4. GONADOTROPINS BLOCKADE.

5. CORTISOL-LIKE ACTIVITY (?).

FIG. 7.   Role of MPA in breast cancer treatment.

dihydrotestosterone binding sites. Abundant evidence supports its antiproliferative
effect on endometrial cancer cells along with a reduced rate of labelled estrogen
uptake by the cell. Moreover, MPA was shown to inhibit estradiol binding to
estradiol specific receptors *in vitro* breast carcinoma (5). There is also a direct
effect, typical of progestins, consisting in MPA inhibition of the replenishment of
the cytoplasmic estrogen receptor; the hypothesis was also made that progesterone
interferes with the nuclear linkage of the estrogen-receptor complex, which would

LOW RISK	HIGH RISK
DISEASE FREEE INTERVAL > 2 yrs.	DISEASE FREE INTERVAL < 2 yrs.
OLDER PATIENTS	YOUNGER PATIENTS
SLOW-GROWTH TUMOR	RAPID-GROWTH TUMOR
LOW-RISK METASTASES:	HIGH-RISK METASTASES:
nodes	lymph vessels
skin	visceral
bone	contralateral breast
single metastasis	multiple sites
pleural effusion	CNS

FIG. 8. Risk groups for unknown-receptors patients.

change the pattern of nuclear synthetic activity usually stimulated by the complex itself. Clearly, this process combines with a reduced sensitivity of target cells to estrogen; that is why, from this point of view, progestational agents and antiestrogens can be said to produce fairly similar effects (2–11,24).

In addition, progestins exert a control function on other hormones (24) by competing for nonspecific hormone receptors, and by regulating incretion and levels of circulating hormones. Their antiandrogenic effect is the result of lowered testosterone plasma levels and increased hepatic androgen-reductase (thereby increasing the rate of androgen catabolism), reducing steroidogenesis by the testes (this probably at high doses only), interacting with androgen receptors, decreasing gonadotropin secretion.

When progestins are assessed on the basis of their influence on the specific endocrine control system in prostatic and mammary carcinoma, it can be said that they produce a protective effect against an androgenic environment, which seems to be an essential event in promoting tumor growth, especially in prostatic cancer.

Besides competing with estrogen for specific estrogen receptors, as mentioned above, progestins produce their antiestrogenic effect by blocking hypophyseal secretion of both gonadotropins, by accelerating enzymatic transformation of estradiol into estrone, thus reducing the length and degree of cell exposure to the action of the most effective estrogen, and by reducing the rate of transformation of androgens into estrogens.

As to their influence on prolactin, progestins reduce the number of prolactin-specific receptors in target cells, and modulate prolactin secretion through the estrogen control. Moreover, it is likely that prolactin may, in turn, control progestin receptor content possibly through an indirect effect; in fact, in experimental breast cancer, the quantity of estrogen receptor, which is an essential factor in the estrogenic stimulation of cell "paving" with progestin receptors, appeared to be dependent on prolactin levels. In humans, pathologic levels of circulating prolactin are apparently influenced by administration of exogenous progestins; however, the rare studies that have been conducted on this effect provided only conflicting and inadequate information for any final conclusion. As to the hypophyseal block induced by progestins, this is a well-known and deeply investigated event: hypophyseal block depresses levels of hypophyseal gonadotropins (with luteinizing hormone decreasing more steadily), decreases adrenocorticotropic hormone levels, and reduces secretion of prolactin through an estrogen-mediated effect. By interfering with secretion of luteinizing hormone, progestins may probably influence the prostaglandin secretion, thereby controlling cell growth and pain, i.e., modifying the cancer cell environment, like antiestrogens (see above).

Progestins compete also for glucocorticoid receptors in mammary cancer cells, and they cause blood hydrocortisone levels to fall. Clinical use for a certain period of time of medium-high dose progestins may cause untoward side effects, such as increased blood sugar levels, hypertension, and a condition quite similar to Cushing's disease. The above clinical and biochemical manifestations are to be accounted for not only by a number of different pathogenic factors but also by the hydrocortisone-like effect produced by MPA, or most likely, its metabolites; in fact, a certain MPA favorable effect on pain was partly ascribed to MPA central and peripheral steroidal action, which is the result of an oxygenated corticoid metabolite of MPA (14).

Finally, an important finding for the clinical application of progestational agents is the amount of protection they provide against bone-marrow toxicity induced by chemotherapeutic agents (30). Controlled studies in which MPA was employed with combination chemotherapy showed that leucopenia was a significantly less serious side effect in hormone-treated patients than in patients receiving chemotherapy alone. The mechanism of action responsible for this drug effect is still being investigated.

In conclusion, MPA is a synthetic steroidal compound with complete progestational activity and many different points of interference on the specific endocrine-modulating complex of some hormone-related tumors (Figs. 6 and 7). MPA acts directly upon cancer cells, and at medium-high doses it may produce a real cytotoxic effect on target cells (31). Indirectly MPA also produces several mediated effects, all of them being related to endocrine physiopathology of breast cancer: these effects include interfering at estrogen receptors level, on the hypothalamic-hypophyseal axis, and with secretion of prolactin, estrogen, and androgen. All of these effects represent the basis of MPA antitumor activity, as well as of its favorable and untoward side effects, as discussed in detail below.

In summary, considering the mechanisms of action of both TAM and MPA, they share a common, but in its nature still different, competitive activity against estrogens and estrogen receptors: whereas the former shows a direct receptor competition with estrogens, the latter inhibits the cell "priming" for estrogen receptors. Therefore, both TAM and MPA are "protecting" against the estrogenic environment favorable to tumor growth. MPA acts at various points within the endocrine control system of the tumor, and is supposed to induce a higher cytotoxic effect at its currently used doses. In addition, MPA also possesses a cortisol-like activity, which is in some ways favorable and in others unfavorable from the therapeutic point of view. Finally, some specific, inherent properties of each drug make the use of each one more or less preferable within the overall therapeutic strategy for mammary carcinoma.

DOSES AND THERAPEUTIC RESPONSE

Considering only controlled studies, featuring sound criteria for response evaluation, the median response rate for TAM is 32% (16–52%) with a response duration of approximately 12 months (8–20). Duration of response has probably been underestimated because of studies still under way and covering too short periods of time. Currently, 20 to 40 mg of TAM are administerd daily by mouth, and plasma levels, as evidence of drug distribution and catabolism, become steady in about 4 weeks. That is why at least 2 months must be allowed prior to assessing TAM for its clinical and biological efficacy. Increasing doses of TAM did not seem to improve significantly response rate and duration. TAM and its demethylated metabolite have fairly long half-lives (7 and 14 days, respectively). This is just preliminary information, and additional investigation is required prior to establishing whether splitting the drug administration over a given period of time may produce the same benefits as mentioned above, with lower doses, respectively. As far as we know, 40 mg/day might be the initial induction dose, while 20 mg/day might be an effective maintenance dose. The comparatively long half-life of TAM must be taken into account when employing TAM in combination with chemotherapeutic agents or other hormones, especially when TAM and other drugs are parts of an alternate, sequential therapeutic strategy. A recent paper reports lower therapeutic efficacy for an antiestrogen–progestin combination than for the antiestrogen alone. This result may possibly be related to a reciprocal interference of the two compounds at receptors level with a resulting depressed specific activity by each of them (17).

Initially, TAM was essentially used to treat postmenopausal patients, and only in recent studies have premenopausal women also been included. However, no significant difference has been noticed between pre- and postmenopausal patients from the therapeutic point of view, despite the fact that a few investigators have reported higher response rates with older patients; in regard to the endocrine modulating system in mammary and endometrial cancer, and specifically to the prevailing estrogenic function favoring tumor growth, there is no aspect on which discrimination between pre- and postmenopausal patients can be based as far as drug efficacy is concerned. The only exception to this is the possibly higher amount of receptor-estrogen complexes in older women; in fact, to produce its effect TAM needs to interact with estrogen receptors. This might also apply, at least conceptually, to highly differentiated and rapidly growing tumors that are less responsive to hormonal manipulation because of their low estrogen receptor content; under this condition, hormonal therapy in conjunction with chemotherapy, or regimens including drugs active on a higher number of sites than TAM, would be more useful.

Concerning metastatic sites, soft tissue metastases appear to be more responsive than skeletal metastases, while only moderate response can be expected from visceral metastases. However, a few investigators have reported satisfactory results with visceral metastases too, but a larger number of cases is necessary to confirm their results. Bone metastases are an interesting subject. In fact, 15–25 percent of patients with osseous metastases respond favorably, and response rate is higher than with high estrogen dosages, and fairly close to the one obtained with progestins.

Data on secondary treatment with TAM of patients who have failed to respond to cytotoxic agents are not numerous in the literature. Several controlled, cross-over studies are now under way. On the basis of available data, we would say that prior treatment with chemotherapeutic agents does not modify the patient's ability to respond to antiestrogen therapy; at the same time, however, a good 50% chance remains that relapses after hormonal therapy may respond to secondary treatment with TAM.

Finally, different attempts were recently made to combine chemotherapy and TAM in programs including one or several chemotherapeutic agents.

Present results are particularly difficult to assess from the point of view of their clinical implications because the number of studies is still relatively small and dating from too short a period of time. However, controlled clinical trials seem to show that a synergic effect is produced by TAM and chemotherapy, as demonstrated by the increase in response rate, which is only rarely significant.

At this moment, no answer can be given about a concomitant, sequential, or alternate schedule of drugs administration, and the possibility of overlapping drug toxicities seems almost negligible.

A deeper insight into these aspects is extremely necessary; in the meantime, we think that combined hormonal chemotherapy should be adopted only for rapidly growing tumors, and whenever other conventional treatment modalities failed.

The possibility that TAM can substitute for ovariectomy in premenopausal women with advanced breast cnacer has also been suggested; of course, TAM does not suppress adrenal androgens conversion into estrogens, but its specific receptor-inhibiting activity may equally reach its main therapeutic objective, that is, to block estrogenic stimulation. It was observed that hypophysectomy can occasionally produce higher response rate than antiestrogens. These increased response rates are most likely the result of a series of alterations induced by hypophysectomy and producing a far-reaching influence within the entire endocrine system. However, on the basis of available information, any interpretation of these alterations would only be speculative. Up to now, we consider that TAM is quite useful in ovariectomized patients as a means of inducing a higher degree of suppression of estrogenic activity.

Untoward effects reported with TAM are of small clinical significance, and only rarely does the drug have to be discontinued. Most patients tolerate the drug well, and only a small number of them report typical untoward effects (hot flushes, vulvar itching, etc.) that commonly accompany estrogen suppression. Gastrointestinal disturbances are generally the cause of treatment discontinuation; however, this occurs in about 3% of patients, and this figure can be lowered by instituting adequate support therapy to reduce gastric secretion, and by controlling the different psychogenic factors that may be involved in individual patients. Another important adverse effect that may be seen during the initial stage of treatment is hypercalcemia, and it may also be accompanied by a more or less high pain increase in subjects with skeletal metastases. However, drug withdrawal, or adequate concomitant medical measures, can lower serum calcium levels, and allow antiestrogen therapy to be resumed. A few authors have correlated increased serum calcium levels and pain to the patient's positivity in estrogen receptors, since they consider hypercalcemia and increased bone pain as evidence of tumor cell sensitivity to hormonal action. In fact, assuming that antiestrogens inhibit prostaglandin synthetase and in view of the fact that prostaglandins are responsible for a certain amount of bone resorption in metastatic osteolysis, then, antiestrogenic compounds should be viewed as a specific and effective therapeutic regimen for this frequent clinical condition in women with advanced mammary carcinoma. Of course, this assumption must be confirmed clinically, and—above all—by significantly higher response rates from osseous metastases than the ones commonly associated with other hormonal treatments. At this moment, reported response rates are quite comparable, despite a small number of studies showing a better percentage trend for TAM. However, differences in experimental conditions and other sources of variance make it hard to say a final word on this subject.

In the 1970s medium-high doses (500–1500 mg/day) of MPA were found to elicit overall response in approximately 40% of patients with metastatic breast cancer, with widely varying rates being reported by individual investigators. Such a broad range of response rates can be accounted for by different criteria used in patient selection (age, metastatic dissemination, previous therapy, etc.), as well as by difference in response evaluation criteria (especially in patients with skeletal lesions).

In recent controlled clinical trials (21–30), a response rate of approximately 40% was reported for a therapeutic regimen employing 500 mg MPA/day. Progressively increasing dosage levels do not substantially improve that rate. In a tentative way, since additional controlled studies are necessary to investigate differences between routes of administration, and to compare the results obtained with moderately low dosage levels, a regimen of 500 mg/day for 30 days, then 500 mg i.m. twice a week until recurrence of the disease can be recommended. Even though pharmacokinetic studies of MPA are still under way, it seems that MPA can slowly reach its plasma steady state after i.m. injection, and that it remains at a steady state for more than 2 weeks. After that period of time, plasma levels of MPA start falling if no additional amount is administered. MPA has a fairly long half-life (about 5 weeks) also on account of its low solubility and slow absorption at the site of injection.

After oral administration of MPA, its plasma peak concentration can be reached in a few hours, and it falls quite rapidly (within approximately 24 hr) when treatment with MPA is discontinued. Oral administration may lead to differences in rates of absorption between individuals, and this may also cause problems in maintaining steady plasma drug levels. Fractionated daily administration might reduce or eliminate this drawback.

MPA has been used mostly in postmenopausal women, and that is why the larger share of available results refer to them. Recently, studies including fertile women have reported rates of response that compare quite favorably with those in postmenopausal patients. It does not seem that the number of years from menopause, or the patient's age, can bring about significant statistical differences.

As to the therapeutic response, it can be said that two important clinical events may appear as early as the initial days of treatment: first, pain, when present, decreases or disappears in about 70–80% of patients. This analgesic effect, which is quite comparable to the one elicited by hypophyseal alcohol injection, cannot yet be accounted for by available information. On the basis of the ability MPA has been demonstrated to possess in blocking secretion of gonadotropins, particularly of luteinizing hormone (24), it may be assumed that MPA interferes via the hypophyseal block on prostaglandin formation. In addition, the analgesic effect observed following MPA administration can in part be the result of the peripheral and central steroidal activity of the drug, since it seems that MPA is catabolized through transformation into an oxygenated steroid (14). The second significant early clinical event is the improvement in the patient's performance status and sense of well-being, which is psychologically beneficial to the patient. This phenomenon is most likely dependent upon a hydrocortisone-like effect of MPA, that is also responsible for other manifestations, as we shall see when discussing side effects of MPA. A high percentage of response from metastases is obtained with soft tissue metastases. Rates of response from bone metastases show a broad range of variation between studies, and frequently reach 50%. Also considering the difficulties in assessing skeletal metastases response, the above percentage, which was also reported for controlled clinical trials (30), is quite a suggestive one. As with antiestrogens, antagonism with prostaglandins might be assumed for progestins too, but in the latter case a completely different mechanism seems to be involved. For instance, blocking hypophyseal secretion of gonadotropins by MPA might interfere with prostaglandin secretion. MPA was also reported to induce anabolism, and this might be the stimulating factor of the synthesis of bone matrix, or the repair process of metastatic skeletal lesions.

As with other hormonal therapies, the rate of response that could be obtained with MPA in two controlled studies featuring a therapeutic strategy based on patients' receptor status was higher. It was demonstrated that antiestrogens and progestational agents produce comparable response rates when response is correlated to hormone receptor levels in tumor cells (30). These data are not numerous at the moment and need to be confirmed, especially because of the high doses of MPA that were used. In fact, there is the possibility that MPA does not act only by binding to its specific cytoplasmic receptors, but also by interfering with other hormone receptors, and through hormone interferences within the endocrine control system of the tumor, which is a possibility that cannot be ruled out with certainty at this moment. Use of MPA as secondary treatment, or when other therapeutic conventional measures have failed, made 25–30% of patients respond, albeit partially and for a relatively short period of time (4,15). This result was obtained both after chemotherapy alone and chemotherapy plus endocrine therapy. It is interesting to mention here that both TAM and MPA showed complete lack of cross-resistance, which means that both of them can be used as secondary treatments. Also MPA was tested in combinations including various chemotherapeutic agents, as described in a recently published review (30).

On the whole, results as to response rates are in favor of hormonal therapy in combination with chemotherapy rather than chemotherapy alone. However, as said when discussing combinations including antiestrogens, many answers must still be given to questions, such as which are the best combinations, the chemotherapeutic regimen and the treatment sequences to be preferred and, above all, which patients are the best candidates for this therapeutic strategy. As to the final question in our series, we hold the view that until better understanding of some essential points is gained, and evidence is obtained that the above type of combined hormone-chemotherapy strategy gives better results than sequential combination therapy and improves the patient's quality of life, it must be considered as strictly experimental. Therefore, it should be adopted only in controlled clinical trials including patients with a rapidly evolving disease, or refractory to other treatments.

Both TAM and MPA can be included as the hormonal constituent in combinations with chemotherapeutic agents. In fact, low incidence of untoward effects is reported for both of them, and they enhance toxicity of concomitant chemotherapy only slightly. As a result of its protective myelosuppression (the mechanism of which has still to be elucidated), and the marked improvement in performance status and sense of well-being induced by MPA, this progestational agent seems to be preferable, although not in an absolute way, over TAM. Side effects are more frequent with MPA than TAM. However, when MPA is employed at medium dosage levels, careful clinical management can prevent side effects from occurring, or reduce their severity without discontinuing therapy. Hyperglycemia is often an expression of preexisting chemical diabetes turned into overt diabetes, while only rarely can this adverse reaction be completely ascribed to a real hydrocortisone-like effect by MPA. However, our own experience and that reported by other investigators indicates that when diabetes is present, and insulin therapy is required, MPA, and especially high doses of it, are contraindicated. Hypertension is reported, particularly in patients over 60 years, or those with preexisting transitory attacks of hypertension or a stabilized form of hypertension. Most likely, increased blood pressure is the consequence of MPA-induced water-salt retention, and of the hydrocortisone-like effect (permissibility with catecholamines?) mentioned above. After prolonged MPA treatment, a Cushing-like syndrome may develop not only in patients receiving high drug doses. Generally, this untoward effect is moderate, and can be overcome by lowering MPA dosage; moreover it is a persisting condition only in a few rare cases. Tremor, sweating, vaginal bleeding, muscle cramps, and phlebothrombosis have been reported occasionally with MPA. However, they could be clinically overcome.

Regarding the above untoward effects, therapeutically advantageous side effects produced by MPA include increasing appetite and body weight (which is very valuable psychologically especially in depressed patients), improved sense of well-being, leukocyte and platelet protection against toxicity caused by chemotherapy, and analgesia. The latter effect was observed by several investigators and was taken as the basis for the use of MPA as an analgesic drug. According to a few investigators, MPA induces an intense pain-relieving effect in about 80% of patients. Even though we have not run any controlled study to investigate this effect, our response rate is lower. In particular, no significant benefit could be obtained in patients with tumors showing no degree of hormone-dependence in whom MPA (up to 1500 mg/day) was employed mainly for pain relief.

THERAPEUTIC STRATEGY

To design an effective therapeutic strategy for treatment of metastatic mammary carcinoma, a series of pharmacological, biological, and clinical criteria must be considered together, even though weighing them on the basis of their specific relative importance. The most important factors to be considered are age and receptor status, i.e., the quantity of estrogen receptors, and possibly the amount of progestin receptors, the degree of risk, clinical conditions independent from cancer, and previous treatments. Any therapeutic strategy must include only extensively tested drugs, i.e., drugs being classified as conventional or standard therapeutic measures and experimental or pilot programs should be adopted only after the disease has become unresponsive to standard therapy. Indications as to the strategy to adopt for each risk group are provided in our tables, both for patients with known receptor status and patients for whom no receptor assay data are available (see Figs. 9–11).

Risk groups (Fig. 8) should be established on the basis of clinical experience, and the most relevant factors to their establishment are the patient's age, length of disease-free interval between primary therapy and first recurrence of disease, rapid tumor growth, and site(s) of metastases.

Obviously, high-risk patients call for a more aggressive therapeutic strategy than low-risk patients, all other clinical conditions being identical. However, an additional, highly discriminating criterion in the assignment of patients to either the low- or high-risk group is their menopausal status.

Adjuvant treatment given at the moment of primary therapy in the integrated therapeutic approach does not seem to influence the results obtained by conventional therapeutic strategies when patients relapse with disseminating metastases. In fact, the 5-year survival rate for patients with recurrent metastatic tumors who received prophylactic post-surgery chemotherapy is quite comparable with the one reported for control patients (28). The situation is more complex for hormonal adjuvant treatment. Here, no adequate evaluation can be made of a few prophylactic hormonal treatments for two reasons: first, trials were run comparing their results with historical data or in patients with unknown receptor status; second, there is no way of affirming that recurrence of disease in patients who were ovariectomized by radiotherapy for prophylactic purpose (with or without concomitant steroid therapy) proves that their neoplastic tissues were unresponsive to hormonal manipulation.

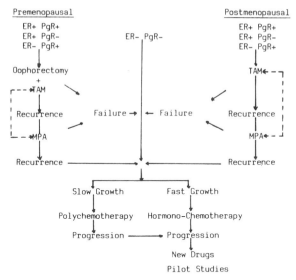

FIG. 9. Treatment strategy in advanced breast cancer: Known-receptors patients.

However, as we have already emphasized, hormonal adjuvant treatment is still an experimental measure, and consequently should not interfere with the selection of the primary treatment to be administered at the time of first recurrence of disease.

As to the study of each patient's receptor status, it is important as it gives better chances to effectively manage the treatment. This applies both to assays of primary tumor cells, and even more to receptor assays performed in metastatic tissue. However, in several investigators' opinion, and in ours, receptor assays should not play a binding role in the selection of the most effective therapeutic strategy. Of course, when the patient's receptor status is known, a more specific therapeutic regimen can be prescribed.

Finally, other factors, such as diabetes, hypertension, cardiovascular disease, and liver disease, may be involved in the selection of the most suitable therapeutic strategy for any cancer patient. All of these factors may increase the risk for the patient, and therefore force the physician to exclude drugs with particularly toxic side effects from the available drug selection. Whenever any of the above complicating factors are involved, chemotherapy should possibly not include drugs producing toxic effects on heart and liver. When similar drugs are essential, their untoward effects should be controlled and minimized as much as possible; moreover, in these particular conditions, antiestrogenic compounds appear to have a wider range of possible applications than progestin, especially as a consequence of the effects elicited by progestins on metabolism and water-electrolyte balance. Since there are no biologically identical individuals, the above evaluation of the two types of hormonal therapy must be part of the decision-making process any physician must go through when selecting a therapeutic strategy for an individual patient. At that moment, his clinical judgement must prevail over every a priori evaluation.

Major steps in our therapeutic strategy for patients with known receptor status are outlined in Fig. 9. Since estrogen is produced in small amounts by the adrenal glands, ovariectomy in conjunction with antiestrogen therapy can be useful in premenopausal women to induce complete estrogen suppression. Also aminoglutethimide can be employed advantageously; however, it is still being investigated, and requires steroidal replacement to be provided under close medical supervision, which is not always feasible for various clinical reasons. Should no response be obtained after a 30–45 day period of treatment, combination chemotherapy should be adopted. In this case, sequential therapeutic programs of proven efficacy should be instituted, using drugs without cross-resistance to each other, or more active chemotherapeutic agents, such as adriamycin, as initial treatment or after relapse.

Should the adopted treatment fail, or in rapidly advancing cancer, contrary to the above considerations, hormone therapy may be adopted in conjunction with combination chemotherapy, and TAM or MPA can be employed alternatively as the hormonal agent. Under this circumstance, the protective effect produced by MPA on bone marrow makes it possible to administer a full-dose chemotherapy and to improve patient's compliance to schedule. That is why MPA appears to be preferable to TAM in this situation. Another consideration in favor of MPA is its ability to improve the patient's general condition, which is often very poor, and reduce pain in patients with rapidly advancing cancer, or already at its advanced stage. Increased appetite and improved sense of well-being, along with its analgesic effect are other favorable side effects produced by MPA that are extremely beneficial to the patient's quality of life.

At the second recurrence of disease after TAM, MPA proves to be effective, and it can produce response from a good number of patients who have become

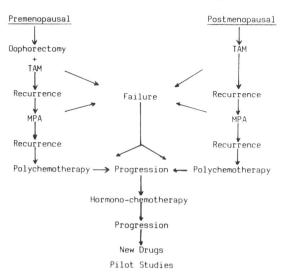

FIG. 10. Treatment strategy in advanced breast cancer: Low risk group of unknown-receptors patients.

unresponsive to other endocrine manipulations. As shown by a dotted line in Fig. 9, the TAM-MPA sequence can be reversed in premenopausal women: in fact the rationale underlying the decision to give TAM first, and MPA as secondary treatment, is to take advantage of the favorable side effects caused by MPA (particularly improved sense of well-being and pain-relief), in patients with more advanced breast cancer in whom more serious clinical conditions are present. However, should pain and the patient's general condition be very severe and manifest after first metastatic growth, no clinical and/or hormonal consideration can oppose the use of MPA as the primary treatment. As a matter of fact, TAM can produce its effects also in patients who failed to respond to prior therapy. In postmenopausal patients, the therapeutic sequence is quite similar, the only exception being ovariectomy. At present, it is our strategy, following endocrine study in every patient who is less than 2 years post-menopausal, to apply castration by radiotherapy in conjunction with antiestrogenic treatment.

In negative-receptor patients, combined chemotherapy is desirable as the primary treatment. However, in patients with rapidly evolving tumors, chemohormonal therapy should be attempted, still in an experimental schedule not only to provide adequate treatment to patients with possible false-negative receptor results, but also in the attempt at taking advantage of the analgesic and protective effects produced by MPA on pain and bone marrow or, respectively, of the specific action produced by TAM on multiple bone lesions (24).

Patients with unknown receptor status are divided into different risk groups, and menopausal status. In the low-risk group (Fig. 10), a treatment sequence very similar to the one we have just described can be employed for similar therapeutic reasons. In high-risk patients (Fig. 11), particularly those under 65 years, chemotherapy should be the primary treatment, and MPA, TAM, and chemotherapy plus endocrine

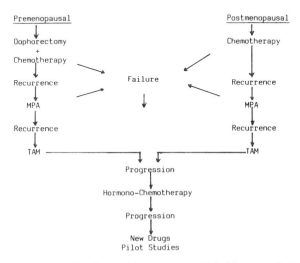

FIG. 11. Treatment strategy in advanced breast cancer: High risk group of unknown-receptors patients.

treatment should follow, in that order, at recurrence of disease. In these patients, the sequence for hormonal therapy is MPA first, TAM second. But this is not strictly binding and the drug sequence can be reversed. It may be suggested that MPA be used first only because its points of attack within the tumor modulating endocrine system are more numerous than with TAM, and therefore it can interfere with a higher number of events favoring cancer cell proliferation.

Finally, a few aspects of the role of hormonal treatment in the adjuvant post-surgical project have to be stressed. Experimental and clinical observations, and in particular the results, although still partly questionable, that have been obtained with postsurgical prophylactic ovariectomy plus cortisol treatment have led hormones and antihormones to be classified as possibly useful ingredients of this integrate cancer therapy; we cannot discuss here some recently published data (16), but prophylactic hormone treatment alone seems to be, under some aspects, aleatory when it is intended to eliminate focal neoplastic lesions that may have been left behind after primary surgery. Suffice it to mention again that hormonal therapy alone is inadequate because both hormone-sensitive and hormone-insensitive cells exist in one tumor, and therefore effective prophylaxis should include both hormones and chemotherapeutic agents, whenever this is possible. When chemohormonal therapy has to be given, the first drug of choice should be the antiestrogenic agent on account of its specific activity within the mechanism of tumoral endocrine control, and its extremely low number of side effects. However, on the basis of receptor assay (essential tool in adjuvant treatment), and a complete study of the patient's endocrine status (including determinations of follicle-stimulating hormone, luteinizing hormone, prostaglandins, prolactin, androgen, etc.), two populations of patients with quite differentiated overall endocrine characteristics may emerge configurating as more convenient to adopt combination chemotherapy plus TAM or MPA in order to provide an individually oriented treatment. But this leads us into a completely experimental field beyond our scope to summarize the criteria on which conventional therapeutic strategy rests.

As stated at the beginning of this chapter, combined hormone regimens are also used in the treatment of metastatic mammary cancer. In this application, combined hormone regimens represent an attempt to take advantage of the endocrine physio-pathologic mechanism involved in hormone-dependent tumors, that is, to interfere with several essential events taking place within the specific endocrine control system, thus bringing tumor proliferation under control. This might lead to new results, reduced drug dosage levels, better use of the mutually potentiating effects of drugs, and less frequent adverse reactions to the treatment. An example of such an attempt is the study of different regimens combining progestins and antiprolactinic agents that was conducted by several investigators (19). Although their results are not final, they are certainly encouraging. Another similar experience is the series of pilot studies of sequential, alternate progestin and estradiol regimens in patients with mammary carcinoma who have become refractory to any conventional treatment (25). The underlying rationale is estrogenic stimulation of progestin receptor replenishment. Overall response from this group of patients totaled 25%, and its duration was approximately 7 months. Since conventional therapy was proven to be no more effective in these patients, the above-reported response rate and duration of response are clearly encouraging, and additional investigational efforts must be made in this area. At present, we are testing an experimental protocol that had already been suggested by us and other investigators (1,23) some time ago. The protocol provides for alternate, sequential courses of treatment with an antiestrogenic compound and a progestational agent in different doses and schedules. Again, the underlying rationale is hormone-receptor stimulation plus the possibility to avoid tumor growth through almost physiologic estradiol dosage levels. Different treatment sequences shall have to be evaluated, and, above all, special consideration shall be given to dosage selection and half-lives for both drugs, and route of administration especially for MPA. All of this is a way of avoiding mutual drug competition, which would clearly imply unfavorable therapeutic results (17).

CONCLUSIONS

TAM and MPA interfere with the specific endocrine control mechanism of mammary carcinoma at partly similar points of the hormonal control system via effects that can be said to be partly similar and partly different. TAM is a major competitor with estrogen for estrogen receptor, and consequently it can influence the level of ambient prolactin and, probably, of gonadotropin. It also inhibits prostaglandin synthetase, which is extremely valuable to patients with bone metastases. As a result of its ability to induce complete estrogen suppression, TAM is employed in ovariectomized premenopausal women, and in combinations with chemotherapeutic agents for prophylaxis (this application is still being tested clinically).

TAM is given as primary treatment instead of MPA to patients with advanced, receptor-positive tumors because MPA is more suitable for the treatment of more severe cases. In fact, it can produce analgesia, increase appetite, and improve the patient's sense of well-being. However, this does not mean that MPA must be used in very serious conditions only, rather, that its administration must be decided upon by the physician for each patient on the basis of several clinical factors.

TAM causes less untoward effects than MPA; however, side effects can also be reduced through careful clinical management during treatment with MPA. When non-tumor-related clinical conditions, such as diabetes, hypertension, and renal failure, are present in patients with advanced breast cancer, TAM is more indicated than high-dose MPA. Theoretically, in patients with advanced breast cancer, MPA should be preferred over TAM as a result of its protective effect against myelosuppression induced by concomitant cytotoxic therapy. However, this cannot be a binding consideration at all, and both drugs can be used, but in a sequential manner immediately after first recurrence of disease.

A particularly interesting feature common to both drugs is their ability to produce a certain amount of response from patients who have failed to respond to other chemohormonal treatments, or have relapsed. TAM is relatively effective after first recurrence of disease in hypophysectomized patients. Special interest has already been generated by studies now being run by several investigators to evaluate the changes caused in receptor concentrations by different therapeutic measures.

Both drugs are clearly not mutually exclusive, or alternative. Each of them plays a fairly well-defined role in each therapeutic strategy for human breast cancer. Actually, as a working hypothesis, or a proposed pilot trial plan, a strategy featuring short, sequential, alternate courses of each drug could be designed to take advantage of each drug-specific stimulation on hormone receptors and its manifold interference with endocrine control of human breast cancer.

Finally, the cost difference between these two drugs, clearly in favor of TAM, should not be an acceptable reason for preferring the antiestrogenic compound to the progestational agent. Actually, the therapeutic value, as well as the improved rate of response and duration of survival, have been documented for both drugs as the result of their rational and sequential use.

Hopefully, their combined use, as allowed by some essential biological variables, will be likely to result in reduced dosage levels, and a treatment regimen that may more closely reflect endocrine physiopathology of human breast cancer.

REFERENCES

1. Bonte, J. (1980): *Hormones and Cancer*, edited by S. Iacobelli, R. G. B. King, H. R. Linder, and M. E. Lippman. Raven Press, New York.
2. Clark, J. H., Anderson, J. N., and Peck, E. J. (1975): *Nature*, 251:446.
3. Clark, J. H., Hsueh, A. J. W., and Peck, E. J. (1977): In: *Biochemical Action on Progesterone and Progestins*, edited by E. Gurpide, p. 161. Academy of Science, New York.
4. De Lena, M., Brambilla, C., Valagussa, P., and Bonadonna, G. (1979): *Cancer Chemother. Pharmacol.*, 2:175.
5. Di Carlo, F., Pacilio, G., and Conti, G. (1975): *Tumori*, 61:501.
6. Ganzina, F. (1979): *Tumori*, 65:563.
7. Gullino, P. (1981): *Angiogenesis Factor and Tumor Progression*. I Annual Meet. Ital. Coop. Oncol. Group, Rome.
8. Henningsen, B., Linder, F., and Steichele, C. (1980): *Endocrine Treatment of Breast Cancer. A New Approach*. Springer-Verlag, Berlin, Heidelberg, New York.
9. Horwitz, K. B., and Mc Guire, W. L. (1978): *J. Biol. Chem.*, 253:8185.
10. Horwitz, K. B., and Mc Guire, W. L. (1980): In: *Endocrine Treatment of Breast Cancer*, edited by B. Henningsen, F. Linder, and C. Steichele, p. 45. Springer-Verlag, Berlin, Heidelberg, New York.
11. Hsueh, A. J. W., Peck, E. J., and Clark, J. H. (1975): *Nature*, 254:337.
12. Iacobelli, S., and Di Marco, A., Eds. (1980): *Role of Medroxyprogesterone in Endocrine Related Tumors*. Raven Press, New York.
13. Jordan, V. C., Naylor, K. E., Dix, C. J., and Prestwich, G. (1980): In: *Endocrine Treatment of Breast Cancer*, edited by B. Henningsen, F. Linder, and C. Steichele, p. 30. Springer-Verlag, Berlin, Heidelberg, New York.
14. Martino, G., and Ventafridda, V. (1976): *Tumori*, 62:93.
15. Mattson, W. (1978): *Acta Radiol. Oncol.*, 17:387.
16. Meakin, J. W. (1980): In: *Endocrine Treatment of Breast Cancer*, edited by B. Henningsen, F. Linder, and C. Steichele, p. 178. Springer-Verlag, Berlin, Heidelberg, New York.
17. Mourisden, H. T., Palshof, T., and Rose, C. (1980): In: *Endocrine Treatment of Breast Cancer*, edited by B. Henningsen, F. Linder, and C. Steichele, p. 169. Spriner-Verlag, Berlin, Heidelberg, New York.
18. Mourisden, H., Palshof, T., Patterson, J.,and Battersby, L. (1978): *Cancer Treat. Rep.*, 2:131.
19. Mussa, A., Dogliotti, L., and Di Carlo, F. (1977): *Min. Med.*, 68:2233.
20. Pannuti, F., Martoni, A., Lenaz, G. R., Piana, E., and Nanni, P. (1978): *Cancer Treat. Rep.*, 62:499.

21. Pannuti, F., Martoni, A., Di Marco, A., Piana, E., Saccani, F., Becchi, G., Mattiolo, G., Barbanti, F., Marra, G. A., Persiani, W., Cacciari, L., Spagnolo, F., Palenzona, D., and Rocchetta, G. (1979): *Europ. J. Cancer*, 15:593.
22. Pellegrini, A.(1981): *Proc. Intl. Symp. on "Role of Tamoxifen in Breast Cancer"*. Raven Press, New York, *in press.*
23. Pellegrini, A., Massidda, B., Mascia, V. (1980): *Proc. Simp. Metastasi Ossee.* Ist. Pascale, Napoli.
24. Pellegrini, A., Massidda, B., Mascia, V., Lippi, M. G., Ionta, M. T., Muggiano, A., and Carboni, E. (1980): In: *Role of Medroxyprogesterone Acetate in Endocrine Related Tumors*, edited by S. Iacobelli and A. Di Marco. Raven Press, New York.
25. Pellegrini, A., Robustelli della Cuna, G., et al. (1981): *Cancer Treat. Rep.*, 65:135.
26. Powles, T. J., Dowsett, M., Easty, D. M., and Neville, A. M. (1981): *Lancet*, I: 608.
27. Ribeiro, G. C. (1977): *Proc. Symp. on Hormonal Aspects of Breast Cancer Therapy*. Tel Aviv.
28. Ritchie, G. A. F. (1980): In: *Endocrine Treatment of Breast Cancer*, edited by B. Henningsen, F. Linder, and C. Steichele, p. 96. Springer-Verlag, Berlin, Heidelberg, New York.
29. Robustelli della Cuna, G., Calciati, A., Bernardo-Strada, M. R., Bumma, C., and Campio, L. (1978): *Tumori*, 64:143.
30. Robustelli della Cuna, G., Pellegrini, A., and Ganzina, F. (1980): *Chemotherapy and Hormonal Treatment of Advanced Breast Cancer*. Farmitalia-Carlo Erba, Milano.
31. Usai, E., Oggianu, F., Ciccu, M., Russino, G., Pinna, A., Ferreli, A., Costa, V., and Pellegrini, A. (1977): *Atti 50° Congresso Soc. Ital. Urol.*, p. 631. Ancona.

Role of Medroxyprogesterone in Endocrine-Related Tumors, Volume II, edited by L. Campio, G. Robustelli Della Cuna, and R. W. Taylor. Raven Press, New York © 1983.

Low- Versus High-Dose Medroxyprogesterone Acetate in the Treatment of Advanced Breast Cancer

*F. Cavalli, **A. Goldhirsch, †F. Jungi,
‡G. Martz, and §P. Alberto For the Swiss Group for
Clinical Cancer Research (SAKK)

*Division of Oncology, Ospedale San Giovanni, 6500 Bellinzona; **Institute for Medical Oncology, Inselspital Bern, 3010 Bern; †Division of Oncology, Medizinische Klinik C., Kantonsspital St. Gallen, 9006 St. Gallen; ‡Division of Oncology, University-Hospital, 8091 Zürich; §Division of Oncology, Hospital Cantonal, 1205 Geneva, Switzerland*

Progestins, and particularly medroxyprogesterone acetate (MPA) have been known for a relatively long time to produce objective tumor regression in women with disseminated breast cancer, and to be practically devoid of severe untoward effects: in the literature the response rate with MPA ranges from 0 to 36% with a tendency to be below 20% in the larger series (5,6,7,10–12). The Swiss Group for Clinical Cancer Research (SAKK) used MPA 500 mg i.m. weekly in a trial comparing chemotherapy versus the combination of chemohormonotherapy. This setting was not particularly suitable for the evaluation of the role of MPA: nevertheless the results seemed to be not only inconclusive, but also somewhat disappointing (1). However, in the last years a renewed interest for MPA in the treatment of advanced breast cancer was prompted by the data published by Pannuti et al. (8) and Robustelli et al. (9), who were able to achieve a response rate above 40% using high dose (1000 mg daily or more) of MPA.

We decided therefore to start a pilot study, in which we treated 19 patients with advanced breast cancer with 1 g daily MPA for 4 weeks (3). The results of this trial (6 partial remissions out of 19 patients) encouraged the SAKK to embark on a randomized trial comparing low- versus high-dose MPA in the treatment of advanced breast cancer. Here we wish to report the *preliminary* results of this trial, which for some subsets of patients has already been closed. As is usual for cooperative groups, many data have still to be reviewed: a final and thorough analysis of the trial is expected to be ready in a few months.

PATIENTS AND METHODS

Patient Selection

All patients selected for this trial had an advanced, measurable breast cancer. In particular, no patient had pleural effusion or osteoblastic bone involvement as the sole clinical evidence of advanced breast cancer. All patients were postmenopausal women. Patients below the age of 65 years were accepted only if they had been pretreated, either with chemotherapy or with an hormonal treatment. Patients above the age of 65 years could enter the protocol, even if previously untreated. Patients with brain metastases, with a performance status >3 (ECOG/SAKK scale) were all excluded from the study.

Between September 1979 and June 1981, 166 postmenopausal women entered into the trial. At the last evaluation of this study (July 1, 1981) 1 patient was too early for a clinical assessment of the antitumor activity (<4 weeks of treatment). Sixteen patients were not evaluable: in nine instances either the patient or the treating physician refused to continue the treatment with the i.m. formulation and switched to an oral MPA treatment. The remaining 7 patients are not evaluable because of early death (<4 weeks after starting the treatment): in most cases those patients had a poorer performance status than that called for by the protocol and could therefore also be listed as protocol violations. Table 1 summarizes the main characteristics of the 149 evaluable patients according to the two treatment schedules (A: 1000 mg daily, B: 500 mg twice weekly). The two treatment groups were fairly comparable in terms of mean age, mean free interval, dominant site of disease, mean number of known metastatic sites, prior therapy, and response to the prior treatment.

TABLE 1. *Pretreatment characteristics of evaluable patients*

MPA Regimen	1000 mg (N = 76)		500 mg (N = 73)	
Mean age (yrs.)	60.9 (40–85)		59.6 (27–83)	
Mean F.I. (mts.)	33.7 (0–185)		28.3 (0–180)	
Dominant site				
locoregional	15	(20%)	12	(16%)
soft-tissue	11	(14%)	12	(16%)
osseous	27	(36%)	25	(35%)
visceral	23	(30%)	24	(33%)
Mean no. of sites	2.2		2.3	
Previous chemotherapy (CT)				
none	15		6	
R to CT	22		24	
NC to CT	6		10	
PD to CT	24		23	
CT not evaluable	9		10	
Previous hormonotherapy (HT)				
none	14		11	
R to HT	25		26	
NC to HT	8		6	
PD to HT	23		25	
HT not evaluable	6		5	

F.I., Free internal; R, response; NC, no change; PD, progressive disease.

Treatment Schedule

Patients were randomized either to regimen A, 1000 mg MPA i.m. daily for 4 weeks except Saturdays and Sundays, or to regimen B, 500 mg i.m. twice weekly for 4 weeks. The protocol called for a treatment of 4 weeks, unless a life-threatening progression occurred earlier. If this was not the case, the patient was evaluated at the end of the 4th week of treatment: patients showing a progressive disease then went off study. Responding patients or those showing at least a stabilization of the disease (no change) received subsequently a maintenance treatment with 500 mg MPA i.m. once weekly. This maintenance treatment was continued until a new progression occurred. For the definition of partial remission (PR), no change (NC), and progression (PD) standard criteria were used (14).

In the course of this trial ancillary pharmacokinetic and endocrinologic studies, which will be reported in details elsewhere, were performed. In 10 patients MPA blood levels were monitored up to the 4th month of treatment: 5 patients were treated with the low, the other five with the high-dose of MPA (13). In the blood samples of 21 patients the following hormones were determined before starting the treatment and 4 and 8 weeks after the beginning of therapy: luteinizing hormone (LH), follicle-stimulating hormone (FSH), prolactin, androstenedione, sex hormone binding globulin (SHBG), cortisol, and E_1 (2).

RESULTS

Table 2 shows the therapeutic results according to the two groups given different dose schedules of MPA. While at this *preliminary* evaluation 20% of the patients show a stabilization of the disease in both treatment arms, the group treated with high-dose MPA shows significantly more remissions (27/76) as compared with the group treated with low-dose MPA (9/73). This difference (35 versus 12%) is statistically significant ($p < 0.01$).

The median time to progression, calculated from the beginning of the treatment, is 393 days for responding patients in regimen A (high-dose MPA), whereas for patients responding to low-dose MPA it is 150+ days. Comparing only the median values, the difference in the time to progression appears to be statistically significant at $p < 0.05$. However, comparing all points of the two curves, there seems to be, at least for the moment, no statistical difference.

TABLE 2. *Therapeutic results*

	No. results / No. of pts. (%)
PR	
1000 mg	27/76 (35%)
500 mg	9/73 (12%)
NC	
1000 mg	16/76 (20%)
500 mg	15/73 (20%)

PR, partial response; NC, no change.

The median survival for all patients treated in this study averages 21 months, whereas for patients progressing under MPA the median survival is around 11 months. Patients responding to the treatment or those showing at least a stabilization of the disease progression have yet to reach the median value of their survival.

Table 3 details the characteristics of the responding patients. Considering the dominant site of the disease, therapeutic responses were achieved mostly in patients having loco-regional, osseous, or soft-tissue lesions. On the contrary, responses were much less frequent in patients with visceral lesions: all responses were furthermore registered in patients presenting lung metastases whereas none of the patients with liver involvement responded to the hormonal treatment.

Comparing the responses by sites, the difference in the remission rate is so far statistically significant between the two treatment groups only in patients with bone metastases as the dominant site of disease. Here 48% (13/27) of the patients treated with high dose of MPA showed a PR, whereas only 8% (2/25) of the cases receiving low-dose MPA registered a similar therapeutic result. However, the differences in the response rate in patients with loco-regional disease and soft-tissue metastases are also striking. Most patients presenting with pain experienced an improvement of this symptom: a more exact evaluation of this point is currently under way. As regards the previous treatment, patients previously nonresponsive to either chemotherapy or hormonal treatment were practically resistant to low-dose MPA, but responded in a remarkable percentage of the cases to high-dose MPA. It is note-

TABLE 3. *Characteristics of responding patients*

Regimen	1000 mg No. resp./No. cases (%)	500 mg No. resp./No. cases (%)
Dominant site		
loco-regional	6/15 (40)	3/12 (25)
soft-tissue	4/11 (36)	1/12 (8)
osseous	13/27 (48)	2/25 (8)
visceral	4/23 (17)	3/24 (12)
	27/76 (35)	9/73 (12)
Previous CT		
none	10/15 (66)	2/6 (33)
R to CT	6/22 (27)	5/24 (20)
NC to CT	0/6 —	0/10 —
PD to CT	6/24 (25)	1/23 (4)
nonevaluable	5/9 (55)	1/10 (10)
Previous HT		
none	9/14 (64)	4/11 (36)
R to HT	10/25 (40)	4/26 (15)
NC to HT	3/8 (37)	0/6 —
PD to HT	5/23 (21)	0/25 —
nonevaluable	0/6 —	1/5 [(20)]

CT, chemotherapy; R, response; NC, no change; PD, progressive disease; HT, hormonotherapy.

worthy that among patients of regimen A there is no clear-cut correlation between the response to MPA and the outcome of the previous hormonal treatment. Patients who hadn't previously received either cytotoxic drugs or an hormonal treatment (and mostly were untreated at all) registered a very high remission rate—around 60% for the group treated with high-dose MPA and around 30% for the group treated with low-dose MPA. It must be noted that almost all of these patients were women above the age of 65 years and mostly showing a slow-growing tumor.

Considering these results, the trial has been closed for previously treated patients, who didn't respond either to the previous chemotherapy or to the hormonal treatment received in the past. The trial is still open for previously untreated patients, and for those who responded to a previous therapy.

Hormonal receptor status of tumors is known in about 30% of the patients, since most of the cases entered into this trial had their mastectomy before the determination of hormone-receptors became a routine procedure in our institutions. Since data regarding the hormonal receptors are still under evaluation, no definite conclusions can be drawn at this moment.

The side effects registered in this trial also have to be further analyzed: however, up to now no major difference has clearly emerged in the pattern of toxicity observed with the two different schedules. Most of the patients demonstrated an increase in body weight in the order of 3–10 kg. Almost all patients noticed a dramatic increase in appetite. Minor vaginal bleeding developed in 3 women, whereas muscle cramps were observed in about 20% of patients during the treatment and for a few weeks thereafter. In about 25% of the patients a median increase of 15–20 mm/Hg in the median value of systolic blood pressure was registered. Up to now we didn't register in our trial any gluteal abscess, a complication which was often reported in previous studies.

DISCUSSION

We present here an interim evaluation of our trial, which for some subsets of patients is still ongoing. It has to be stressed that our current results must still be regarded as preliminary. In fact within the setting of a cooperative group, most data can be definitely assessed only when the final evaluation is performed. This final assessment normally requires an extramural review of at least some cases. Keeping these facts in mind, our preliminary data suggest that high doses of MPA yield superior results in the treatment of advanced breast cancer when compared with the low, conventional MPA dosage.

In trials encompassing an hormonal treatment for advanced breast cancer, differences in the published results often reflect patient selection (age, extent of disease, prior therapy) as well as different criteria for the assessment of the therapeutic results and conflicting methods of reporting data. It is therefore not surprising, that the response rate for the treatment with conventional dose of MPA in breast cancer ranged in the literature from 0 to 36%.

Our preliminary data are consistent with those published by De Lena et al. (4). In fact, in their prospective but not randomized trial, MPA induced an objective tumor response in about 30% of patients. This finding correlates rather well with our 35% remission rate in the treatment group with high-dose MPA. In the Milan trial all patients were heavily pretreated, while in our study about 20% of the women were without previous therapy: this can account for some differences. Moreover, in his paper De Lena stated that: "The patients with a disease-free interval of longer than 2 years, who were postmenopausal and had lesions either in the soft tissue or in the lung and pleura were the ones who benefitted most from treatment with MPA." Whereas in his study one-quarter of the patients were premenopausal, all the women entered in our trial were postmenopausal. Another factor, that explains the favorable response of our cases is the fact that patients above 65 years of age were allowed to enter the study even if not pretreated. In a cooperative setting this means practically that treating physicians were entering into this hormonal trial mainly older patients (and this fact is reflected by the median age of the treated population) with rather slow-growing tumors. De Lena et al. failed to observe a difference in the therapeutic activity between 500 mg i.m. daily × 30 days and 1000 mg i.m. daily × 30 days. Since the schedule used in our study (1000 mg i.m. daily × 5 days per week during 4 weeks) gives, if calculated on a daily base for 1 month, an average daily dosage of about 700 mg, we may well understand why the results of both trials are so similar. Considering the data reported in the literature, the rather disappointing results obtained in our group treated with low-dose MPA cannot be considered fully inconsistent. Of particular interest is the fact that we failed to observe responses with the low treatment in patients, who were primarily resistant to a previous therapy. On the contrary, patients treated with the high dose of MPA responded quite frequently, even if they were previously considered to be nonresponders. This fact is again consistent with the findings of De Lena, who reported a 32% response rate for patients nonresponding to a previous hormonal treatment and a 21% response rate for women previously resistant to cytotoxic drugs.

Noteworthy also is the fact that for the time being we have not been able to detect a major difference in the pattern of toxicity emerging from the two treatment groups. However, a more detailed analysis of the observed side effects has still to be performed. The toxicity registered in our trial is similar to the one reported in earlier studies: however, for the time being we failed to register cases of gluteal abscess.

It is possible that in the future a more appropriate place for progestational agents in the palliative therapy of mammary carcinoma will be found, when hormone receptors are available in all patients at the time of therapeutic decision. Even if in our trial only about one-third of the patients had their hormone receptors determined, we hope that the evaluation of these data will shed some light on this problem.

In conclusion, we feel that for the time being it is very difficult to decide whether high-dose MPA or tamoxifen should be considered as the first treatment of choice in postmenopausal women with such characteristics that lend themselves to a trial of hormonal manipulation. A randomized trial between the two treatments followed by a crossover therapy upon failure appears therefore to be indicated in postmenopausal women with positive or unknown receptors and no hepatic involvement.

REFERENCES

1. Brunner, K. W., Sonntag, R. W., Alberto, P., Senn, H. J., Martz, G., Obrecht, P., and Maurice, P. (1977): *Cancer*, 39:2923.
2. Campana, A., Eppenberger, U., Andor, J., Kaplan, E., Kaplan, S., and Cavalli, F. Endocrinologic evaluation during the treatment of patients with advanced breast cancer with high and low dose of MPA. *Oncology (in press)*.
3. Castiglione, M., and Cavalli, F. (1980): *Schweiz. Med. Wschr.*, 110:1973.
4. De Lena, M., Brambilla, C., Valagussa, P., and Bonadonna, G. (1979): *Cancer Chemother. Pharmacol.*, 2:175.
5. Goldenberg, I. S. (1969): *Cancer*, 23:109.
6. Klassen, D. J., Rapp, E. E., and Hirte, W. E. (1976): *Cancer Treat. Rep.*, 60:251.
7. Muggia, F. M., Cassileth, P. A., Ochoa, M., Jr., Flatow, F. A., Gellhorn, A., and Hyman, G. A. (1968): *Ann. Intern. Med.*, 68:328.
8. Pannuti, F., Martoni, A., Lenaz, C. R., Piana, E., and Nanni, P. (1978): *Cancer Treat. Rep.*, 62:504.
9. Robustelli Della Cuna, G., Calciati, A., Bernardo Strada, M. R., Bumma, C., and Campio, L. (1978): *Tumori*, 64:143.
10. Segaloff, A., Cuningham, M., Rice, B. F., and Weeth, J. B. (1967): *Cancer*, 20:1673.
11. Stoll, B. A. (1966): *Med. J. Aust.*, 1:331.
12. Stoll, B. A. (1967): *Br. Med. J.*, II:338.
13. Tamassia, V., Battaglia, A., Ganzina, F., Isetta, A. M., Sacchetti, G., Cavalli, F., Goldhirsch, A., Kiser, J., Bernardo, G., and Robustelli Della Cuna, G. (1982): Pharmacokinetic approach to the selection of dose schedules of Medroxyprogesterone acetate in clinical oncology. *Cancer Chemother. Pharmacol.* 8:151.
14. WHO Handbook for reporting results of cancer treatment. (1979): WHO, Geneva.

Role of Medroxyprogesterone in Endocrine-
Related Tumors, Volume II, edited by L.
Campio, G. Robustelli Della Cuna, and R. W.
Taylor. Raven Press, New York © 1983.

Medroxyprogesterone Acetate at Two Different High Doses for the Treatment of Advanced Breast Cancer

H. Cortés Funes, *P. L. Madrigal, *G. Perez Mangas, and C. Mendiola

*Hospital "1° de Octubre," and *Hospital Oncológico Provincial, Madrid, Spain*

Medroxyprogesterone acetate (MPA) is a synthetic steroid derived from progesterone and synthesized in 1958 by two different research groups (2,14). Experimental pharmacology data show that MPA is a steroid endowed with a specific progestational action, similar to the physiological action of progesterone, and active both by the oral and intramuscular route of administration. MPA is devoid of estrogenic action (13,14) but exerts antiestrogenic, antiandrogenic, and antigonatropic effects (5) and inhibits conception by blocking ovulation.

MPA acts through multiple mechanisms still under evaluation, such as pituitary blockade, interaction with tumor cell receptors, inhibition of estrogen binding to its receptor, lowering of estradiol levels increasing catabolism and decreasing androgen-estrogen conversion, and inhibiting cellular DNA synthesis with a direct antitumor effect (4). MPA therefore appears, with antiestrogens, as one of the best available additive hormonal treatments for advanced breast cancer (11).

A few years ago MPA was reevaluated as a drug effective in advanced breast cancer, and high doses up to 500 mg were reported to give a 42% and 65% response rate in premenopausal and postmenopausal women, respectively (10). More recently two randomized studies suggested that the ideal dosage lies around 500 mg daily for at least 30 days followed by the same dose two or three times a week indefinitely (9,12), with a response rate of 41%. Another study with the same dose gave only 28% of responses in patients already resistant to chemotherapy (6). Median duration of these responses ranged from 8 to 12 months (6,8,12).

In order to confirm these results, we developed a clinical trial in two different institutions, whose purpose has been an attempt to know the overall response rate, median duration of responses, and toxicity of two different high doses of MPA in women with metastatic mammary cancer. In this chapter we report the results of this study.

PATIENTS AND METHODS

In this study we included patients with metastatic breast cancer mainly resistant to conventional chemotherapy and/or hormonotherapy. Eligibility criteria include pre- and postmenopausal women with measurable and/or evaluable metastasis, survival expectation of up to 3 months, and Karnofsky's performance status up to 50%. Patients were treated in two institutions with doses of 500 and 1000 mg of MPA. Treatment was followed daily i.m. for 30 consecutive days. After this induction period, responding patients continued treatment at the same dosage twice a week until relapse. Characteristics of both groups are detailed in Table 1.

Despite the fact that patients were not randomized the two groups were comparable according to dominant site of metastasis, previous therapy, menopausal status, and age. There was a small difference of 6 months in the median disease-free interval.

Patients started treatment either with 500 or 1000 mg and if there was no progressive disease detectable after 1 month of therapy, the treatment was continued in the same way twice weekly until progressive disease or relapse was detected. When a progressive disease was documented a new treatment, in relation to previous therapy used, was administered.

The results were estimated every fourth week for 12 weeks by means of physical examination, assessment of Karnofsky's index, chest X-ray, and laboratory examination (CBC and SMAC). Bone and liver isotope scans were repeated every 3 months. Estrogen and progesterone receptors were performed in some patients by the charcoal method, but they were not used for the analysis of responses.

Response criteria were the usual for this disease. Complete remission (CR) is the disappearance of all disease, including the radiological recalcification of lytic bone lesions. Partial remission (PR) is more than 50% in the decrease of measurable

TABLE 1. *Patients' characteristics*

	MPA (500 mg)	MPA (1000 mg)	Total
No. of patients	46	43	89
Median age (years)	56	59	57.5
No. of premenopausal patients	15	10	25
No. of postmenopausal patients	31	33	64
Disease-free interval (months)	31	25	28
Dominant site			
soft tissues	22	20	42
visceral	7	8	15
osseous	12	12	24
others	5	3	8
Previous treatment			
chemotherapy alone	11	8	19
hormonotherapy alone	8	9	17
chemo plus hormono	18	14	32
none	9	12	21

lesions and objective improvement in evaluable but nonmeasurable lesions if no new lesions occur. Stabilization or no change (NC) is recorded when the lesions are unchanged (less than 50% but more than 25% of disease of measurable lesions). The subjective improvement was also analyzed but was not included into responses. Progressive disease (PD) is recorded when some lesions regress while others progress or new lesions appear, or when some or all lesions progress and/or new lesions appear. The duration of remission and survival are recorded from the day therapy started.

RESULTS

The analysis of results did not reveal any significant difference between the two treatment groups. Twenty-eight patients (31.5%) show objective responses with 6 (6.7%) complete and 22 (25%) partial remission (Table 2). Global response was a little lower (28%) in patients treated with 500 mg when compared with patients treated with 1000 mg (35%), with more than double of complete responses; this difference was not significant. An additional 30 and 26% of stabilization of the disease was obtained in each group of patients, respectively.

The analysis of responses by dominant metastatic site is detailed in Table 3. There were also no significant differences between the two groups in any subclasses of patients. In patients with soft tissue lesions, the overall percentage of response was 18 and 25%, respectively. In those with prevalent osseous lesions the rate of response was 50% for both groups of patients, and in the group with dominant visceral lesions there was a small difference in favor of the higher dosage with 37 against 28%. In premenopausal patients the response was 16%, lower than in postmenopausal patients, which was 37%. Furthermore there were no differences in the average duration of remission in all subclasses of patients in both groups of dosage (range 2–23 months).

Table 4 shows the analysis of subjective remission. It is important to note the significant reduction of pain in 58/89 (65%) of the cases. This effect is more intensive in patients receiving 1000 mg (77%) than in patients receiving 500 mg (54%). The rest of subjective responses were very similar in both groups of patients.

Responses in relation to previous treatment are analyzed in Table 5. Response rate is somewhat higher in patients without prior therapy (38%) in comparison with

TABLE 2. *Results*

	MPA (500 mg)	MPA (1000 mg)
Complete remission	2 (4%)	4 (9%)
Partial remission	11 (24%)	11 (25%)
Global response	13 (28%)	15 (35%)
No change	14 (30%)	11 (26%)
Progression	19 (41%)	17 (39%)

Numbers in parentheses represent the percentages of the patients treated.

TABLE 3. *Response by metastatic site*

Metastatic site	No.	MPA 500 mg			No.	MPA 1000 mg		
		CR + PR	NC	P		CR + PR	NC	P
Soft tissues	22	1 3 (18%)	9 (41%)	9 (41%)	20	2 3 (25%)	7 (35%)	8 (40%)
Visceral	7	— 2 (28%)	2 (28.5%)	3 (43%)	8	1 2 (37%)	2 (25%)	3 (37%)
Osseous	12	1 5 (50%)	3 (25%)	3 (25%)	12	1 5 (50%)	2 (17%)	4 (33%)
Others	5	— 1 (28%)	—	4 (80%)	3	— 1 (33%)	—	2 (67%)
Total	46	2 11 (28%)	14 (30%)	19 (41%)	43	4 11 (35%)	11 (26%)	17 (39%)

TABLE 4. *Subjective response*

	MPA (500 mg)	MPA (1000 mg)
Relief of pain	25/46 (54%)	33/43 (77%)
Asthenia	18/46 (39%)	19/43 (44%)
Anorexia	24/46 (52%)	24/43 (56%)
PS Impairment	17/46 (37%)	18/43 (42%)
Weight increase	31/46 (67%)	31/43 (72%)

TABLE 5. *Response in relation to previous treatment*

Prior therapy	No.	Response to prior therapy	Response to MPA (CR + PR)
Hormonotherapy (castration, antiandrogens, androgens, estrogens)	17	22%	6 (35%)
Chemotherapy (CMF—CMFVP—CAF)	19	48%	6 (31%)
Hormono plus chemo	32	47%	8 (25%)
None	21	—	8 (38%)
Total	89	—	28 (31.5%)

those previously treated with chemotherapy (31%), hormonotherapy (35%), or both (25%). MPA does not appear to show cross-resistance with these treatments. Median duration of response was 6.8 months with no difference in both regimens, 7.3 and 6.4 months, respectively.

Clinical toxicity connected with the treatment is shown in Table 6. There was no difference in the incidence of side effects in both groups of patients. Gluteal abscess was the only one which limited the continuation of the treatment, present

TABLE 6. *Toxicity*

	MPA (500 mg)	MPA (1000 mg)
Gluteal abscess	10%	11%
Sweating	12%	13%
Cushing facies	17%	19%
Tremor	13%	12%
Cramps	7%	8%
Vaginal bleeding	6%	7%
Thrombophlebitis	2%	0%

in 10 and 11% of patients, respectively. Other toxic effects such as facies lunaris, sweating, tremor, and cramps are acceptable and reversible.

DISCUSSION

MPA has been shown as an effective drug in advanced breast cancer. At low dosage (less than 500 mg/day) the response had never exceeded the 25% of objective remission. In 1972 several investigators began studies on the use of different higher doses equal to or greater than 500 mg/day. The maximum tolerable dose was identified at 1500 mg/day i.m. for 30 days (10). Objective remission with these higher doses ranged from 30 to 50%. This difference was due to several factors which were analyzed in studies done during recent years.

Some of these factors are the level of higher dosage used, the relation to previous therapy, menopausal status, and response criteria used. In relation to the level of dosage to be used, there are two important randomized studies done by Robustelli and Pannuti. The first one (12) compared daily dosage of 500 with 1000 mg on 101 postmenopausal women not previously treated with chemotherapy. There was no difference between response rates in both groups of patients: 43% of patients showed objective remission, with 44% response rate in the group of 500 mg/day and 41% with the 1000 mg/day regimen. In this trial skeletal and soft tissue metastasis were the localization with best response. The mean duration of response was 8 and 9 months for each regimen, respectively.

In the other study Pannuti et al. (9) randomized 92 patients to receive MPA 500 or 1500 mg/day i.m. for 30 days. These patients were also not treated previously with combination chemotherapy. The response rate was 44% with no significant difference between both regimens (43 and 54%, respectively). However, differences were noted in regard to side effects. The 500-mg/day regimen had fewer side effects with better tolerance.

Three other investigators studied the antitumor effect of high dosage MPA in patients previously treated with chemotherapy, obtaining lower objective remission. De Lena (3) treated 81 patients with a two-dose schedule of MPA in a nonrandomized study. Objective remission was obtained in 21% of patients treated with 1500 mg/day and 32% on patients treated with 1000 mg/day. Median duration of response was 5 and 7.5 months, respectively.

Amadori et al. (1) treated 74 patients with a dose of 1000 mg/day and obtained a 45% objective remission. All patients were postmenopausal relapsing from previous combination chemotherapy and hormonotherapy. In a group of 25 previously treated breast cancer patients, studies by Mattson (6) with 1000 mg/day obtained a 28% remission with a median duration of 5 + months.

In our original study we obtained a 22% remission in a group of 27 heavily pretreated patients with a median duration of response of 6.5 months (7). In the present study we try to know the influence of previous therapies in another group of patients treated with 1000 mg/day and compare the results with a similar group of patients treated at the standard high dose of 500 mg/day. The global response rate of this study is slightly higher (31.5%) than the previous one, due, probably, to a better performance status of the patients. There was a predominance of soft tissue metastases (48%) in relation to other localization (26% osseous and 16% visceral). This fact could also explain the lower response rate obtained in this study in relation to the previously mentioned studies of Robustelli and Pannuti. The global response of patients treated with 1000 mg/day was higher (35%) than that of patients treated with 500 mg/day (28%), with 9 and 4% complete remission, respectively. Though this difference is not significant, the subjective improvements are much better for the higher dosage group, with special attention to pain relief.

The analysis of response in relation to previous treatment shows that patients responding to hormonotherapy have a better response rate (35%) than patients treated with chemotherapy alone or combined with hormonotherapy (25%). Patients not previously treated have the best response rate (38%).

The last factor of influence in response rate obtained with high dosage MPA is menopausal status. As in the case of other hormonotherapies, premenopausal patients are less responsive to MPA than postmenopausal.

On the basis of these data and the analysis of literature we can conclude that high doses of MPA produce a good objective response rate in patients with advanced breast cancer. This response has a direct relation to the localization of metastasis, previous treatment, and menopausal status, and no relation to the dosage when it was above 500 mg. This fact is not true in relation to subjective improvement of patients with special attention to pain. Dosages of 1000 mg/day produce the same response rate with a better analgesic effect than 500 mg/day, with the same incidence of side effects. Future studies with combination chemotherapy or other hormonotherapy will further clarify the exact role of MPA in the management of advanced breast cancer.

REFERENCES

1. Amadori, D., Ravaioli, A., and Barbanti, F. (1976): *Min. Med.*, 1–4.
2. Babcock, Y. V., Gutselle, S., Heve, N. H., Hogg, Y. A., Stucky, Y. C., and Barnes, W. E. (1958): *J. Am. Chem. Soc.*, 80:2904.
3. De Lena, M., Brambilla, C., Valagussa, P., and Bonadonna, G. (1959): *Chemother. Pharmacol.*, 2:175–180.
4. Di Marco, A. (1980): In: *Role of Medroxyprogesterone in Endocrine-Related Tumors*, edited by S. Jacobelli and A. Di Marco, p. 1. Raven Press, New York.

5. Ganzina, F. (1979): *Tumori*, 65:563–585.
6. Mattson, W. (1978): *Acta Radiol. Oncol.*, 17(5):387.
7. Mendiola, C., Mañas, A., Ramos, A., Quiben, R., Moyano, A., and Cortes Funes, H. (1979): *Oncología*, 80(3):21–26.
8. Nenci, I. (1978): *Cancer Res.*, 38:4204–4207.
9. Pannuti, F., Martoni, A., Di Marco, A. R., Piana, E., Saccani, F., Becchi, G., Mattioli, G., Barbanti, F., Cacciari, L., Spagnolo, F., Persiani, W., Mazza, G. A., Palenzona, L., and Rocchetta, D. (1979): *Europ. J. Cancer*, 15:593–601.
10. Pannuti, F., Martoni, A., Lenaz, G. R., Piana, E., and Nanni, P. (1976): In: *Functional Exploration in Senology*, European Press, Ghent, Belgium.
11. Pellegrini, A., Massidda, B., Mascia, V., Lippi, M. G., Ionta, M. T., Muggiano, A., and Carboni-Boi, E. (1980): In: *Role of Medroxyprogesterone in Endocrine-Related Tumors*, edited by S. Jacobelli and A. Di Marco, p. 29. Raven Press, New York.
12. Robustelli Della Cuna, G., Calciati, S., Bernardo-Strada, M. R., Bumma, C., and Campio, L. (1978): *Tumori*, 64:143–150.
13. Sala, G. (1960): *Annali di Ostetricia e Ginecologia*, 82(4):322.
14. Sala, G., Baldratti, G., and Arcari, G. (1958): *Acta Endocrinol. (Kbh)*, 29:508.

Role of Medroxyprogesterone in Endocrine-
Related Tumors, Volume II, edited by L.
Campio, G. Robustelli Della Cuna, and R. W.
Taylor. Raven Press, New York © 1983.

High-Dose Medroxyprogesterone Acetate in Metastatic Breast Cancer: Preliminary Report on Three AIO Phase II Trials

H. -E. Wander, H. -H. Bartsch, **H.-Ch. Blossey,
and G. A. Nagel

*Department of Internal Medicine, Division of Hematology and Oncology and **Division
of Endocrinology, University of Goettingen, D-3400 Goettingen,
Federal Republic of Germany*

Medroxyprogesterone acetate (MPA) has been reported to induce remissions in breast cancer. Observations that this effect is dose-dependent and at high MPA doses not receptor-specific have stimulated considerable interest in the reevaluation of the role of MPA in the treatment of metastatic breast cancer. The current knowledge has been summarized elsewhere (4) and in this volume.

Whereas sufficient data have been accumulated to prove the efficacy of high-dose MPA as a single agent, experience with high-dose MPA in combination chemotherapy regimens is limited. For this reason the Association of Interdisciplinary Oncology (AIO) activated a series of Phase II studies in order to explore promising chemotherapy/MPA combinations which are suitable and safe for phase II trials. Preliminary data on these trials are presented here.

MITOMYCIN C AND MPA

Mitomycin C (MMC) like MPA is one of the drugs currently reevaluated for the treatment of metastatic breast cancer (3). There are four multicenter trials including MMC listed in the current compilation of experimental cancer therapy protocol summaries (2) and several other trials are under way at individual institutions.

The place of MMC in the hierarchy of drugs against breast cancer has not yet been defined. The current protocol was started aiming at the development of effective third-line drug regimens after more conventional therapies have failed. The combination of MMC and MAP was chosen because both agents are easily administered and subjectively well tolerated even by patients with far-advanced symptomatic breast cancer.

The MPA dose was 500 mg p.o. three times daily throughout the study. MMC was given at a dose of 4 mg/m^2 daily as 3 hr short time infusion for 5 days from day 1 to 5 and 15 to 19 of each cycle. Cycles were repeated every 3–5 weeks.

Thus a total dose of 40 mg/m^2 MMC was given per cycle. In order to allow the evaluation of the therapeutic effectiveness of the drug combination the criteria of patient eligibility for response evaluation were as follows: progressive disease after use of first- and second-line chemotherapy, minimal life expectancy of 2 months, no concomitant tumor therapy, and minimum one course of chemotherapy completed. It was left to the investigators, however, to enter additional patients into the protocol who did not meet the entry criteria of the protocol. Such patients were evaluated for toxicity only.

The characteristics of the patients treated in the protocol are listed in Table 1. Seventy-four patients were evaluated for toxicity and 46 for treatment response. As seen in Table 1, all patients were heavily pretreated with multiple drugs and the majority of them had both postoperative irradiation as well as multiple organ

TABLE 1.   *MMC and MPA: Patient characteristics of the trial*

	Patients evaluated for side effects (N = 74)	Patients evaluated for therapeutic effects (N = 46)
Age (years)		
median	54.8	55.2
range	31.6–77.2	35.0–76.2
Menopausal status		
pre	28	17
peri	5	3
post	41	26
Karnofsky status		
median	62	57
range	20–90	20–90
Site of lesion		
soft tissue	2	2
bone	13	9
lung	6	5
mixed sites	53	30
Prior therapy		
mastectomy	73	46
postop. radiation	65	41
Prior chemotherapy		
adriamycin	37	27
cyclophosphamide	49	32
vincristine	36	24
methotrexate	49	35
trofosfamide	18	14
5-fluorouracil	45	30
Prior endocrine therapy		
oophorectomy	17	12
radiomenolysis	12	7
androgens	15	10
estrogens	14	10
anti-estrogens	48	30
progesterone	7	4
prednisone	22	16

involvement with tumor. About 80% of the patients demonstrated hematologic side effects which are moderate secondary to MMC and to be analyzed elsewhere. It is remarkable, however, that only 6 patients had platelet counts that dropped to 100.000 and below, and only 4 patients showed incomplete recovery of platelet counts despite permanent MMC withdrawal. There is strong evidence that hematologic toxicity of MMC was reduced by MPA. This observation, however, needs substantiation by a prospective trial.

The nonhematological side effects are summarized in Table 2. Weight increase, tremor, edema, and Cushingoid syndrome are side effects clearly related to MPA. There were two side effects which, on the basis of the literature, we did not expect in such frequency and severity—namely lung and kidney toxicities.

In about 50% of the cases dyspnea appeared or increased. Only 5 patients had a decrease of dyspnea following therapy. The pulmonary condition of 3 patients deteriorated to such an extent that artificial respiration became necessary. Sixteen patients' chest X-rays showed signs typical for an interstitial lung process. Histological examination of the lung tissue was done in 4 patients. In 3 patients there was alveolitis and/or fibrosis of the lung; in 1 patient carcinomatous lymphangitis only. Although we have no exact pathologic proof of the lung changes in the other patients, we must suspect drug-induced pneumopathy in some of the other cases not biopsied. The reason is that some lung changes and/or dyspnea developed even if there was evidence of a tumor remission and that symptoms in some patients improved after MMC withdrawal. At this point we are left with the following questions:

1. Is the unusually high incidence of pulmonary toxicity related to MMC only or is it a combination effect of the two drugs involved? MPA given as a single drug does—to the best of our knowledge—cause pulmonary changes only indirectly by cardiac insufficiency or lung embolism but not by direct local lung toxicity.

TABLE 2. *MMC-MPA: nonhematological side effects*
(N = 74)

Side effect	Patients (N)	Patients (%)
Weight increase	40	54
Dyspnea (new + increase)	39	52
Pulmonary densities	16	22
Creatinine elevation	11	15
Tremor	8	11
Edema	8	11
Skin necrosis	5	7
Nausea	5	7
Cushing syndrome	5	7
Hemolytic uremic syndrome	4	5
Lung fibrosis	3	4

2. What roles do drugs play that were previously given in the development of these lung complications?

Further studies are needed to answer these questions.

The second unforeseen toxicity was hemolytic uremic syndrome (HUS), which developed in 4 patients. The potential nephrotoxicity of MMC was first described by Liu et al. (5) in 1971. Fifteen percent of our patients showed increase in creatinine which did not return to normal. Four of these patients developed acute renal failure with hemolytic crises. Histologic evaluation of kidneys in 3 patients demonstrated microangiopathic lesions. Again, we are left with the question whether the addition of MPA to MMC has contributed to this extraordinarily frequent severe kidney toxicity.

The therapeutic results of the study are given in Table 3. The overall response rate was 50%, which is unexpectedly high considering that these were all far-advanced, pretreated, negatively selected cases. There was no remarkable difference in the site of response. Fifty percent of the patients suffering from bone pain secondary to metastases experienced relief of pain even if there was no evidence of tumor remission. The endocrine receptor status was available in 4 patients only. One patient with a positive estrogen and progesterone receptor status showed a partial remission lasting 4 months. Estrogen, progesterone, and androgen receptors were negative in the remaining 3 patients and these did not respond to the treatment with MMC and MPA. As demonstrated in Fig. 1, median survival of responders was 10.5 months versus 5.9 months for nonresponders. Studies to further analyze the possible synergistic effects of both MMC and MPA and the exact frequency of pulmonary changes of both drugs are currently in process.

TABLE 3.   *MMC-MPA: Therapeutic results*

	CR	PR	NC	PD
No. of patients	2	12	9	23
Duration of response (weeks)				
mean	—	21	16	—
range	16/26	7–40	7–23	
Site:				
soft tissue	1	5	4	—
bone	1	2	8	—
lung	1	5	5	—
liver	—	1	—	—
Median survival (months)		10.5	5.9	
Menopause				
pre	—	2	3	10
peri	—	—	2	1
post	2	10	4	12
Median duration CT (days)	123	129	125	78
Median total dose MMC	172	157	150	85

CR, complete remission; PR, partial remission; NC, no change; PD, progressive disease; CT, chemotherapy.

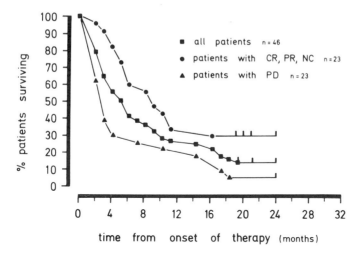

FIG. 1. Mitomycin C and MPA in metastatic breast cancer; Patients survival from onset of therapy.

VINCRISTINE/ADRIAMYCIN/CYTOXANE AND MPA

In another protocol of the AIO we are currently evaluating the combination of vincristine (V) administered at a dosage of 1 mg/m^2 i.v. on day 1, adriamycin (A) administered at a dosage of 40 mg/m^2 i.v. on day 1, cytoxane (C) administered at a dosage of 200 mg/m^2 per os on days 3 to 6 (repeated every 3–4 weeks) and MPA (1500 mg daily per os). This protocol is a feasibility study for a planned phase III protocol comparing different treatment strategies with these four drugs. We are able to present preliminary data on 36 patients who have been treated in Goettingen. All patients received at least three cycles of VAC-MPA. A comparison of data obtained in this study is made with results from a similar patient group reported by others (8), who treated their patients with VAC only. Patient characteristics are presented in Table 4. Although there are more postmenopausal women in our protocol, poor prognostic factors dominate: more patients had a low performance status and 50% of the patients were in relapse after prior chemotherapy.

Furthermore—as summarized in Table 5—in our study 25 out of 36 patients presented with additional poor prognostic factors. The treatment results of these protocols are given in Table 6. Less than 10% of the patients did not respond to the treatment. Of the group of 18 women not pretreated 17/18 had either complete remission, partial remission, or disease stabilization. Only one report in the literature allows for comparison of toxicity data of high- and low-dose MPA in combination with chemotherapy (9). As judged from these data (Table 7) high-dose MPA compared with low-dose does not result in an increased MPA toxicity. Three patients in our study developed symptoms of cardiotoxicity requiring adriamycin withdrawal. Again, with this chemotherapy-MPA-drug combination there is evidence of improved bone marrow tolerance. Under a previous treatment with CMF 5 patients

TABLE 4. *Patient characteristics of 2 VAC protocols*

Characteristic	VAC (Rainey) N = Patients	VAC-MPA (Wander) N = Patients
Patients	32	36
Age		
mean	57	56
range	30–79	28–71
Free interval		
<1 yr	14	16
1–5 yr	14	15
>5 yr	4	5
Menopause		
pre	14	6
post	18	30
Karnofsky		
60+	27	18
<60	5	18
Previous chemo-therapy	0	18

TABLE 5. *VAC-MPA: Poor prognostic factors*

Familial breast cancer	9
Hyperprolactinemia	8
Familial breast cancer + cystic disease	1
Familial breast cancer + hyperprolactinemia	5
Cystic disease + hyperprolactinemia	2
	25/36 Patients

TABLE 6. *Treatment results of two VAC-protocols*

	VAC		VAC-MPA			
			Total		No prior CT	
	w/32	%	n/36	%	n/18	%
CR	9	28	5	14	5	28
PR	14	44	10	28	7	39
NC ⎤	9	28	18	50	5	27
PD ⎦			3	8	1	4

CR, complete remission; PR, partial remission; NC, no change; PD, progressive disease; CT, chemotherapy.

TABLE 7. *Side effects of two MPA protocols*

Characteristics	FAC-MPA, 500 mg p.o. ($N = 40$)	VAC-MPA, 1500 mg p.o. ($N = 36$)
Hair loss	33	35
Mucositis	5	1
Cystitis	3	0
Cardiotoxicity	0	3
Moon facies	2	7
Muscle cramps	4	6
Vaginal bleeding	4	0
Thrombophlebitis	2	0
Increased		
blood pressure	4	3
body weight	22	17
perform-status	18	22
Pain relief	18	18

developed bone marrow toxicity which called for dose modifications. When treated with VAC-MPA these patients showed no significant changes in complete blood count.

AMINOGLUTETHIMIDE AND MPA

The aims of the third AIO protocol are the following:

to develop combination regimens of different hormones;
to determine the therapeutic activity and side effects of aminoglutethimide (AG) and MPA;
to measure hormone and MPA blood levels under these regimens and
to relate results to prognostic variables of the disease;
and finally to evaluate whether MPA could replace cortisone which is given together with AG.

AG has a proven activity in metastatic breast cancer (1). AG was administered at a dosage of 1000 mg/day per os (this dosage was reached gradually within 2 weeks) and MPA was generally administered at a dosage of 1500 mg/day. This evaluation relates only to patients treated by the group in Goettingen. Some of the patients' characteristics are given in Table 8. They indicate that a rather unfavorable group of patients was selected. Endocrine data of this trial are not yet fully evaluated. Suffice it to say that hyperprolactinemia, which generally goes along with a poor prognosis in breast cancer (7), developed in 7 patients treated with AG-MPA.

The side effects of this drug combination are given in Table 9, indicating that their type and frequency were as expected from the literature. Since both drugs might induce hypothyroidism respective symptoms must be carefully looked for. About one-third of the patients lost weight despite the massive MPA doses. An

TABLE 8.   *AG-MPA: Poor prognostic factors*

1.	Familial breast cancer	4
2.	Hyperprolactinemia	10
3.	Second primary tumor	1
	Combination of 1–3 + cystic disease	6
7.	Patients developed HPRL under treatment with AG-MPA	21/29
	Previous hormonal treatment	6
	Previous chemotherapy	8
	Previous hormonal + chemotherapy	15

TABLE 9.   *AG + MPA: Side effects (N + 29)*

Symptom	Expected (%)	AG-MPA Protocol (%)
Vertigo[a]	30–40	34
Drowsiness[a]	30–40	45
Ataxia[a]	30–40	34
Skin eruption	15–30	24
Hypothyroidism	<5	5
Leucopenia	<5	5
Weight increase	20–30	10
Weight loss	<5	28
Obstipation	—	17

[a]First 3 weeks of treatment.

TABLE 10.   *AG-MPA: Therapeutic results*

Result	N Patients	
CR	—	
PR	1 ⎤	
MC	13 ⎬	21/29
NC	7 ⎦	
P	4 ⎤	
Early loss (erythema)	1 ⎬	8/29
Too early for evaluation	3 ⎦	

CR, complete remission; PR, partial remission; NC, no change.

explanation for this observation is expected after endocrine data have been evaluated. Therapeutic results of the trial are presented in Table 10. No complete remission was noted. The explanation is that most patients presented with lytic bone disease, which by definition must be recalcified in order to qualify for complete remission (CR) classification. The response rate with AG and MPA is slightly over 60%.

CONCLUSIONS

On the basis of the data available by our group and other authors (4,6) the following interim judgements can be made on the use of MPA in combination chemotherapy:

1. MPA appears to be a hormone that is particularly suitable for combination chemotherapy regimens because of its high therapeutical efficacy and its anabolic effects which compensate for unwanted side effects of cytotoxic chemotherapy.

2. The high response rates and the low hematological toxicity observed in phase II combination chemotherapy–MPA trials especially in heavily pretreated patients justify further phase III trials. Such studies would prove whether chemotherapy and MPA is more effective and less toxic than chemotherapy alone.

3. On the other hand, it is quite possible that the combination of chemotherapy with MPA results in an increase not only of remissions but also of given side effects of chemotherapeutic agents. Particularly the effects of MPA on connective tissues, water balance, mucous membranes, and epitheliae might be important, for instance on drug distribution in body fluids or drug penetration through membranes. The relatively high interstitial pulmonary toxicity we have seen with MMC-MPA might be the result of such drug interactions. Accordingly, it will be essential in trials with chemotherapy and high-dose MPA to carefully monitor cardiac, pulmonary, kidney, and endocrine functions, particularly if the drugs involved have such organs as toxicity targets.

4. Another important aspect in combination chemotherapy–MPA regimens will be the absorption of MPA given p.o. when drugs toxic to mucous membranes of the gut are involved. Obviously there exist considerable individual and interindividual differences in MPA absorption. Drugs toxic to the gut might further influence enteral MPA uptake.

REFERENCES

1. Ashbury, R. F., Bakemeier, R. F., Fölsch, E., McCune, C. S., Savlov, E., and Bennett, J. M. (1981): *Cancer*, 47:1954–1958.
2. *Compilation of Experimental Cancer Therapy Protocol Summaries* (1981): U.S. Department of Health and Human Services, NCI, Washington.
3. De Lena, M., Jirillo, A., Brambilla, C., and Villa, S. (1980): *Tumori*, 66:481–487.
4. Iacobelli, S., Longo, P., Scambia, G., Natoli, V., and Sacco, F. (1980): In: *Progress in Cancer Research and Therapy, Vol. 15*, edited by S. Iacobelli and A. di Marco, pp. 97–106. Raven Press, New York.
5. Lui, K., Mittelman, H., Sproal, E. E., and Elia, E. G. (1971): *Cancer*, 28:1314–1320.
6. Mattsson, W. (1978): *Acta Radiol. Oncol.*, 17:387–400.
7. Nagel, G. A., Wander, H. -E., and Blossey, H. -Ch.: *Schweiz. Med. Wschr. (in press)*.
8. Rainey, J. M., Jones, S. E., and Salmon, S. E. (1979): *Cancer*, 43:66–71.
9. Robustelli della Cuna, G., and Bernardo-Strada, M. R. (1980): In: *Progress in Cancer Research and Therapy, Vol. 15*, edited by S. Iacobelli and A. di Marco, pp. 53–64. Raven Press, New York.

Role of Medroxyprogesterone in Endocrine-
Related Tumors, Volume II, edited by L.
Campio, G. Robustelli Della Cuna, and R. W.
Taylor. Raven Press, New York © 1983.

The Results of Treatment with Medroxyprogesterone Acetate at High and Very High Doses in 237 Metastatic Breast Cancer Patients in Postmenopause

F. Pannuti, M. R. A. Gentili, A. R. Di Marco, A. Martoni,
M. E. Giambiasi, R. Battistoni, *C. M. Camaggi, P. Burroni,
E. Strocchi, G. Iafelice, E. Piana, and **G. Murari

*Divisione di Oncologia, Ospedale M. Malpighi, 40138 Bologna; *Istituto di Chimica Organica, Università degli Studi di Bologna, 40136 Bologna; **Istituto di Farmacologia, Università degli Studi di Bologna, 40126 Bologna, Italy*

In 1973 we proved that medroxyprogesterone acetate (MPA) could be administered in high doses (15,17) and that the maximum dose tolerable was 1500 mg/i.m./day, for a minimum of 30 days. Subsequently, we and other authors have administered high-dose MPA ($\geqslant$500 mg/i.m./day) for at least 30 days in the treatment of advanced breast, prostate, and kidney cancer (1,2,4,7,11,13,16,18). We also showed that it could be administered orally at high doses (12). Oral and intramuscular high-dose MPA has a powerful anabolizing and analgestic effect (1,10,12). In this chapter we will summarize the conclusions drawn from such experiments on the use of oral and intramuscular high-dose MPA in the treatment of advanced breast cancer from 1973 up to today.

MATERIALS AND METHODS

The study concerns 205 postmenopausal women affected by advanced breast cancer, whose life expectancy is greater than 2 months, and who have normal heart, kidney, and liver functions. They had not undergone any oncological treatment for at least a month prior to this study and had not previously been treated with a high dose ($\geqslant$500 mg/day) of MPA. Histological test confirmed the existence of cancer in these patients. Further clinical tests demonstrated the progressive deterioration of the patients' conditions at the onset of the treatment. The patients' qualifying statistics are listed in Table 1.

MPA was administered intramuscularly for 30 days, to three groups of patients, according to the following daily doses: 500, 1500, and 2000 mg. The intramuscular treatment was terminated after 1 month, due to the high incidence of local intolerance

TABLE 1. *High doses of MPA in metastatic breast cancer: Data on treated patients*

	Intramuscular (mg)			Oral	
	500	1500	2000	2000 mg	Totals
No. of pts.	47	97	17	44	205
Age					
< 50 yrs	7	25	4	9	45
50–60 yrs	15	33	5	12	65
61–70 yrs	18	28	4	20	70
> 70 yrs	7	11	4	3	25
Time from menopause					
1–5 yrs	14	36	6	17	73
>5–10 yrs	10	28	2	12	52
>10 yrs	23	33	9	15	80
Free interval					
0 yrs	6	9	2	3	20
≤2 yrs	25	49	6	13	93
>2 yrs	16	39	9	28	92
Performance status					
30–50%	16	51	12	12	91
60–70%	19	22	5	18	64
80–100%	12	24	0	14	50
Dominant metastatic sites[a]					
ST	10	19	2	10	41
O	26	44	9	25	104
V	11	34	6	9	60
C.I. (V/ST + O)	0.305	0.539	0.545	0.257	0.414
Previous systemic treatment					
oophorectomy:					
prophylactic	8	12	2	5	27
therapeutic	0	11	3	2	16
androgens	9	15	4	0	28
progestagens	2	3	0	2	7
estrogens	1	2	0	0	3
antiestrogens	0	0	0	17	17
chemotherapy:					
adjuvant	3	5	1	2	11
therapeutic	11	12	2	2	27

[a]ST, soft tissue; O, osseous; V, visceral; C.I., comparative index.

(gluteal infiltrate and abscess). As of yet, no maintenance regimen has been established to test the possible latent side effects of this treatment. A fourth group of patients was treated orally with high-dose MPA (2000 mg/day for 30 days) and underwent a maintenance therapy consisting of 1000 mg/os/day until either tolerance or progression was attained.

No antitumor therapy was administered either during or after the treatment. For at least 3 months after the treatment the patients were given monthly clinical examination. In addition, each patient's response to the treatment was evaluated by radiographic examination at 1-, 3-, and 6-month intervals. The evaluation criteria were as follows: CR (complete response), complete disappearance of all lesions for at least 6 months; PR (partial response), the reduction, for at least 1 month, of at least 50% of all measurable lesions' surface area, or, in the case of osseous metastases, the absence of change or the thickening of lesions coupled with the remission of pain for at least 3 months; MR (minimal response), a decrease (ranging between 25 and 50%) in the surface area of all measurable lesions for at least 1 month; NC (no change), no appreciable change or no more than a 25% increase in measurable lesions; P (progression), a 25% increase in at least one measurable lesion, the occurrence of new lesions, or the progression of osteolitic metastases.

All the patients have been continuously and regularly checked until the present or until exitus. Those patients showing progression underwent a polychemotherapy (CMF), while those who suffered recurrence after CR, PR, MR, or NC, underwent either another cycle of MPA, or antiestrogen treatment followed by polychemotherapy.

RESULTS

The side effects of i.m. and oral therapy are recorded in Table 2 according to dose and the manner of administration.

We conclude that: (a) the toxicological aspects of this wider study are similar to those we observed in our first studies on this subject (15–17) and to those observed by other authors (3,11,20,21); (b) aside from localized intolerance problems, the toxicological profile observed after oral administration is identical to that observed after intramuscular administration. All symptoms spontaneously reverted after a short time (within 1–2 months after suspension of treatment).

Table 3 shows the pharmacodynamic responses of the patients who have been separated according to the dominant lesions. The total remission rate (CR + PR) is 40%, and as high as 48% if we consider CR + PR + MR. Patients with bone metastases show a better remission rate (56%).

Table 4 shows the patients' responses to both routes of administration and different dose levels. The best therapeutical results (greater remission rate and smaller pro-

TABLE 2. *High doses of MPA in metastatic breast cancer: Side effects*

Side effects	Intramuscular (mg)			Oral 2000 mg (%)
	500 (%)	1500 (%)	2000 (%)	
Abscess	1 (2)	25 (26)	1 (6)	—
Gluteal infiltration	1 (2)	4 (4)	2 (12)	—
Facies lunaris	3 (7)	10 (10)	4 (24)	—
Acne	—	2 (2)	—	—
Sweating	1 (2)	6 (6)	4 (24)	9 (20)
Fine tremors	—	14 (15)	3 (18)	9 (20)
Cramps	1 (2)	11 (11)	—	8 (18)
Vaginal spotting	—	11 (11)	1 (6)	7 (16)
Methrorragia	—	—	—	1 (2)
Itching	—	1 (1)	—	4 (9)
Insomnia	1 (2)	2 (2)	—	3 (7)
Constipation	1 (2)	—	—	3 (7)
Thrombophlebitis	—	1 (1)	—	3 (7)

The numbers in parentheses represent the percentages of patients treated.

TABLE 3. *High doses of MPA in metastatic breast cancer: Results according
to dominant metastatic lesion*

Dominant metastatic lesion[a]	No. of pts.	Response to therapy[b]				
		CR (%)	PR (%)	MR (%)	NC (%)	P (%)
ST	41	2 (5)	13 (32)	3 (7)	11 (27)	12 (29)
O	104	—	58 (56)	2 (2)	16 (15)	28 (27)
V	60	—	9 (15)	12 (20)	15 (25)	24 (40)
Totals	205	2 (1)	80 (39)	17 (8)	42 (20)	64 (31)

[a]ST, soft tissue; O, osseous; V, visceral.
[b]The numbers in parentheses represent the percentages of patients treated.
CR, complete response; PR, partial response; MR, minimal response; P, progression; NC, no change.

TABLE 4. *High doses of MPA in metastatic breast cancer: Results according to
different schedules*

MPA doses	No. of pts.	Response to therapy[a]				
		CR (%)	PR (%)	MR (%)	NC (%)	P (%)
500 mg i.m.	47	1 (2)	18 (38)	2 (4)	7 (15)	19 (40)
1500 mg i.m.	97	1 (1)	40 (41)	11 (10)	20 (20)	25 (26)
2000 mg i.m.	17	—	7 (41)	1 (6)	4 (24)	5 (29)
2000 mg os	44	—	15% (34)	3 (7)	11 (25)	15 (34)
Totals	205	2 (1)	80 (39)	17 (8)	42 (20)	64 (31)

[a]The numbers in parentheses represent the percentages of patients treated. CR, complete response; PR, partial response; MR, minimal response; P, progression; NC, no change.

gression rate) are demonstrated by the 1500 mg/i.m. group, and the lowest by the group treated orally, although these differences are not statistically significant.

The percentage of objective responses (CR + PR) was also analyzed and compared among the patients according to their age, amount of time after menopause, duration of free interval and, finally, performance status. The results (test X^2) show no statistically significant difference between the various subgroups.

It should be pointed out, however, that those patients with a free interval of more than 2 years tend to show a higher remission percentage than those with shorter free interval. Similarly, patients in menopause from more than 10 years show a higher remission rate (34/80, 43%) than those in menopause from 5 to 10 years (18/52, 35%), or less than 5 years (30/73, 41%). Apparently, there is a reverse correlation between age and remission rates: patients under 50 years of age (20/45, 44%); patients between 50 and 60 years of age (24/65, 37%); patients between 61 and 60 years of age (30/70, 43%), and patients over 70 years of age (8/25, 32%). Finally, those patients with a performance status between 30% and 50% before treatment show a greater response rate (39/91, 43%) than both those with a performance status between 60 and 70% (24/64, 38%), and those between 80 and 100% (19/50, 38%).

Table 5 shows the difference in results according to the patients' previous treatments. The best responses, even if the differences are not statistically significant, are in the "no previous treatment" group and in the "hormone-treated" group.

As far as the median duration of remission is concerned, this was longest in the group of patients affected by osseous metastasis (7.7 months, ranging between 3 and 51 months). Taking into consideration the dosage schedule and the way of administration, the duration of remission was longest in patients treated with 2000 mg/day by intramuscular route (9.5 months) and shortest in those treated by the oral route (5.5 months).

The positive effect of the treatment (at different doses and routes of administration) on particular signal symptoms is shown in Table 6. Although the best responses are shown by MPA 1500 mg/i.m./day, the difference is not statistically significant.

The high effectiveness of the MPA treatment on pain and anorexia is of notable importance. The body weight of 155 patients has also been recorded before and after the treatment; the results show that there was an increase in 91/155 (59%)

TABLE 5. *High doses of MPA in metastatic breast cancer: Results according to previous treatments*

Previous treatment	No of pts.	Response to therapy[a]				
		CR (%)	PR (%)	MR (%)	NC (%)	P (%)
Chemo-hormone therapy	36	0	13 (36)	4 (11)	6 (17)	13 (36)
Hormone therapy	67	1 (2)	28 (42)	8 (12)	13 (19)	17 (25)
No treatment	102	1 (1)	39 (38)	5 (5)	23 (23)	34 (33)
Totals	205	3 (1)	90 (44)	17 (8)	42 (20)	64 (31)

[a]The numbers in parentheses represent the percentages of patients treated. CR, complete response; PR, partial response; MR, minimal response; P, progression; NC, no change.

TABLE 6. *High doses of MPA in metastatic breast cancer: Subjective remission according to different schedules*

Symptoms	MPA Dosages[a]				
	500 i.m.	1500 i.m.	2000 i.m.	2000 os	Total (%)
Pain	21/29 (72)	57/65 (88)	11/13 (85)	15/24 (63)	104/131 (79)
Dyspnea	4/9 (44)	21/31 (68)	2/4 (50)	3/14 (21)	30/58 (52)
Asthenia	17/25 (68)	48/66 (73)	5/11 (45)	8/16 (60)	78/118 (66)
Anorexia	12/15 (80)	34/40 (85)	10/12 (83)	9/12 (75)	65/79 (82)
Walking impairment	4/10 (40)	24/36 (67)	3/4 (75)	6/15 (40)	37/65 (57)

[a]The numbers in parentheses represent the percentages of patients treated.

patients after the treatment (mean increase of 2.5 kg). Also the performance status measured according to Karnofsky improved after high-dose MPA treatment in 94/157 (60%) cases.

Figure 1 shows graphically the 48-month survival period (actuarial analysis) of the patients according to their varying responses to treatment: we can see a significant improvement in CR + PR, MR and NC over P, and of CR + PR over NC. Figure 2 correlates the patients' survival period with their previous treatments. The "no previous treatment" group responded significantly better than the groups pretreated with chemo- and/or hormone therapy.

OUR PRESENT EXPERIENCE AND FUTURE PERSPECTIVES

As the side effects of oral high-dose MPA administration (2000 mg/day) have been shown to be negligible, our experience has demonstrated this drug's clinical efficiency. Consequently, we have decided to administer the drug at higher doses in order to determine the maximum level tolerated without serious side effects. Such a study will also gauge the limits of the clinical usefulness of this drug.

This particular study involves 32 patients affected by advanced breast cancer whose life expectancy is greater than 2 months and who have normal heart, kidney, and liver functions. None of these patients had undergone any oncological treatment for at least a month before the onset of the MPA treatment. Histological test

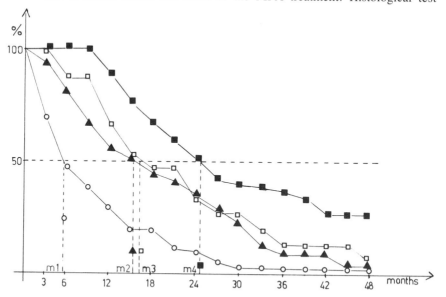

FIG. 1. Survival according to response. *Filled squares:* CR (complete response) + PR (partial response) (79 pts.); median (m4) = 24.6 months. *Open squares:* MR (minimal response) (15 pts.); median (m3) = 16.6 months. *Triangles:* NC (no change) (39 pts.); median (m2) = 15.6 months. *Circles:* P (progression) (59 pts.); median (m1) = 5.9 months. Statistically significant comparisons: CR + PR → NC, $p < 0.01$; CR + PR → P, $p < 0.01$; MR → P, $p < 0.01$; NC → P, $p < 0.01$.

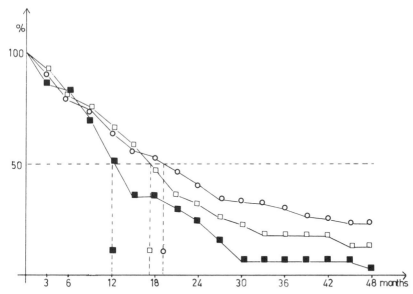

FIG. 2. Survival according to previous treatments. *Circles:* No previous treatment; median (m3) = 19.3 months. *Filled squares:* Previous hormone therapy; median (m2) = 17.6 months. *Open squares:* Previous chemotherapy; median (m1) = 12 months. Statistically significant comparison: No previous treatment → previous chemotherapy, $p < 0.05$.

confirmed the existence of cancer and further clinical tests demonstrated the progressive deterioration of the patients' conditions at the outset of the treatment.

MPA was administered according to the following schedules: (a) 3000 mg/day for 60 days, then 2000 mg/day until tolerance or progression was attained (8 patients); (b) 4000 mg/day for 60 days, then 3000 mg/day until tolerance or progression was attained (13 patients); (c) 5000 mg/day for 30 days, then 4000 mg/day until tolerance or progression was attained (19 patients). The evaluation criteria and the follow-up models are the same as used in the previous study.

The side effects observed in 32 evaluable patients are shown in Table 7. The results are highly similar to those observed in the previous study using lower dosages. These symptoms were not important, since they reverted spontaneously after a short time (within 1–2 months after the suspension of the treatment).

Table 8 shows the objective responses according to the dose level. For the combined responses (CR + PR + MR) the total remission rate is 50%. The high percentage of objective responses apparent in the 4000-mg group can be explained by the smaller number of patients with visceral metastases in this group as compared with the 3000- and 5000-mg groups. The increase of body weight and the improvement of performance status reported in these patients confirm the anabolizing and analgesic effect of MPA found in previous studies (14,21). The same signal symptoms as before were registered initially and 1 month after the treatment (Table 9). Once again this drug proved to be highly effective with regard to pain and anorexia.

TABLE 7. *High oral doses of MPA in metastatic breast cancer (3000–4000–5000 mg/day/os): Side effects*

Fine tremors	8/32 (25)
Cramps	3/32 (9)
Cushingoid aspect	1/32 (3)
Constipation	1/32 (3)
Nausea	1/32 (3)
Sweating	1/32 (3)
Dyspepsia	2/32 (7)

The numbers in parentheses represent the percentages of patients treated.

TABLE 8. *High oral doses of MPA in metastatic breast cancer (3000–4000–5000 mg/day/os): Objective response*

Dose	CR (%)	PR (%)	MR (%)	Total responses	P (%)	NC (%)
3000	0/6	0/6	0/6	0/6	4/6 (66)	2/6 (33)
4000	1/12 (8)	9/12 (75)	0/12	10/12 (83)	0/12	2/12 (16)
5000	0/14	5/14 (35)	1/14 (7)	6/14 (38)	5/14 (35)	3/14 (21)
Total	1/32 (3)	14/32 (43)	1/32 (3)	16/32 (50)	9/32 (28)	7/32 (22)

The numbers in parentheses represent the percentages of patients treated. CR, complete response; PR, partial response; MR, minimal response; P, progression; NC, no change.

TABLE 9. *High oral doses of MPA in metastatic breast cancer (3000–4000–5000 mg/day/os): Subjective response*

Symptoms	3000 (%)	4000 (%)	5000 (%)	Totals (%)
Pain	4/7 (42)	3/7 (43)	9/11 (81)	16/25 (64)
Asthenia	3/8 (37)	3/6 (50)	4/8 (50)	10/22 (49)
Anorexia	4/5 (80)	3/4 (75)	4/7 (57)	11/16 (68)
Walking impairment	0/1	2/5 (40)	0/7	2/13 (15)
Dyspnea	1/3 (33)	0/1	3/4 (75)	4/8 (50)

The numbers in parentheses represent the percentages of patients treated.

The comparison of biochemical parameters before and after 1 month of treatment shows that there is no significant difference except in the case of WBC (as already shown) and BUN (however, within normal values).

CONCLUSIONS

The enlargement of our case study of advanced breast cancer postmenopausal patients treated with high-dose MPA confirmed the results found in 1973 and 1974 (15,17). These data are also confirmed by others (5,6,8,9,22) demonstrating that MPA is particularly suited to these patients.

The remission rates of several groups of patients (with no previous treatments, and with bone or soft tissue metastases) are among the highest rates obtainable with any kind of hormone therapy. The use of modern criteria (e.g., level of hormone receptors) will most likely improve these results. Oral doses of 2000 mg/day tend to show inferior results with respect to those obtained with the corresponding intramuscular dose. The difference in pharmacokinetics of MPA found when administered orally or intramuscularly probably explains this discrepancy. In fact, after i.m. administration, MPA plasma levels are not very high, but persistent for a long period; while after oral administration, they rapidly reach a peak of high maximum and sharp decrease. Preliminary pharmacokinetic data from a study now in progress at our Institute exemplify this process. Clearly, these data raise problems as to the optimum dose, mode of administration, and method required to maintain the drug at clinically effective plasma levels for long periods. Although the solution to these questions is not yet known, it can be safely stated that high-dose MPA objectively and subjectively controls metastatic breast cancer and can be used as a first choice treatment together (simultaneously or subsequently) with chemotherapy (14,19,21). Moreover, we can conclude that daily administrations using as much as 5000 mg of MPA have not yet reached the maximum tolerated dose, since the side effects are similar to those we obtained with lower dosages (21). Clinically, the results of these dosages appear to be superior to those obtained at a dose level of 2000 mg (21), but a statistical comparison between these results is not possible, given the features of this study. Therefore, a statement on the possible advantages of higher doses must be confirmed by further study.

REFERENCES

1. Amadori, D., Ravaioli, A., and Barbanti, F. (1976): *Minerva Med.*, 67:1.
2. Amadori, D., Ravaioli, A., Rodolfi, R., Tonelli, B., Gentilini, P., Casadei, A., Verdecchia, G., Barbanti, F., Dell'Amore, D., and Gardini, G. (1979): *Chemiot. Oncol.*, 1:44–49.
3. Bernardo Strada, M. R., Imparato, E., Aspesi, G., Pavesi, L., and Robustelli Della Cuna, G. (1980): *Minerva Med.*, 1–6.
4. Bumma, C., and Di Carlo, F. (1979): *Boll. Soc. Piem. Chirurgia, IL*, 3:327–336.
5. Cooperative Breast Cancer Group (1961): *Cancer Chemother. Rep.*, 11:109–141.
6. Cooperative Breast Cancer Group (1964): *Cancer Chemother. Rep. (Suppl. I)*, 41:1–24.
7. De Lena, M., Brambilla, C., Valagussa, P., and Bonadonna, G. (1979): *Cancer Chemother. Pharmacol.*, 2:175–180.
8. Goldenberg, I. S. (1969): *Cancer*, 23:109–112.
9. Klaassen, D. J., Rapp, E. F., and Hirte, W. E. (1976): *Cancer Treat. Rep.*, 60:251–253.
10. Martino, G., and Ventafridda, V. (1976): *Tumori*, 62:93–98.
11. Mattsson, W. (1978): *Acta Radiol. Oncol.*, 17(5):387.
12. Pannuti, F., Fruet, F., Piana, E., and Strocchi, E. (1978): *IRCS Med. Sci.*, 6:118.
13. Pannuti, F., Martoni, A., and Cricca, A. (1978): *IRCS*, 6:177.
14. Pannuti, F., Martoni, A., Di Marco, A. R., Rossi, A. P., Fruet, F., Strocchi, E., Lelli, G., Burroni, P., Pollutri, E., Marraro, D., and Piana, E. (1979): *Boll. Soc. Piem. Chir.*, II(3):275–290.
15. Pannuti, F., Martoni, A., Lenaz, G. R., Piana, E., and Nanni, P. (1976): In: *Functional Explorations in Senology*, edited by C. Colin, P. Franchimont, W. Gordenne, P. Juret, R. Lambotte, J. Lavigne, G. F. Leroux, B. A. Stoll, and R. Vokaer, p. 253. European Press, Ghent, Belgium.
16. Pannuti, F., Martoni, A., Lenaz, G. R., Piana, E., and Nanni, P. (1978): *Cancer Treat. Rep.*, 62:499.

17. Pannuti, F., Martoni, A., Pollutri, E., Camera, P., Losinno, F., and Giusti, H. (1976): *Panminerva Med.*, 18:129.
18. Pannuti, F., Rossi, A. P., and Piana, E. (luglio 1977): *IRCS*, 5:375.
19. Pellegrini, A., Massidda, B., Mascia, V., Pasqualucci, S., Desogus, A., and Manni, A. (1978): *Proceed. XII Int. Cancer Congr., Buenos Aires*, Abstr. 10-W 47.
20. Robustelli Della Cuna, G., Bernardo Strada, M. R., Calciati, A., Bumma, C., and Campio, L. (1978): *Tumori*, 64:143–150.
21. Robustelli Della Cuna, G., Martinetti, L., Bernardo Strada, M. R., and Pizzamiglio, D. (1978): *Proceed. XII Int. Cancer Congr., Buenos Aires*, Abstr. 3.
22. Segaloff, A., Cuningham, M., Rice, B. F., and Weeth, J. B. (1967): *Cancer*, 20:1673–1678.

Role of Medroxyprogesterone in Endocrine-
Related Tumors, Volume II, edited by L.
Campio, G. Robustelli Della Cuna, and R. W.
Taylor. Raven Press, New York © 1983.

Oral or Intramuscular Treatment of Advanced Breast Cancer with Medroxyprogesterone Acetate: A Review

J. Løber, H. T. Mouridsen, and C. Rose

Department of Oncology A, Finsen Institute, Copenhagen, Denmark

The overall response rate in metastatic breast cancer patients treated with endocrine therapy is approximately 30%. In recent years it has been recognized that a response to endocrine therapy can be predicted in approximately 60% of the cases, provided that the patients' tumor tissue contains the estrogen receptor (ER) protein (38).

Progestins given at pharmacological doses have been tested for antitumor activity in patients with metastatic breast cancer since the mid 1950s (11,12). Medroxyprogesterone acetate (MPA: 17-hydroxy-6α-methyl-pregn-4-ene-3,20-dione, 17 acetate), a synthetic C-21 progestin, was developed in 1958 and shortly thereafter became the most commonly used progestagen agent for treatment of advanced breast cancer.

POSSIBLE MODE OF ACTION OF MPA AT THE CELLULAR LEVEL

In some experimental mammary tumor models, progestins alone have been shown to promote tumor growth (26,27). However, given in combination with estrogen progestins the drug can both induce tumor regression (27) and prevent tumor appearance (37). In human mammary tumors it also seems that some endogenous estrogen is necessary to obtain tumor regression by treatment with progestins (66).

The mode of action by which pharmacological doses of MPA lead to tumor regression is largely unknown. As is the case with other progestins, MPA lowers the circulating levels of luteinizing hormone (LH) and follicle-stimulating hormone (FSH) (58) and thereby decreases the estrogen concentration in the blood. Furthermore, MPA reduces the plasma cortisol concentration, probably by suppressing adrenocorticotropic hormone (ACTH) secretion (22).

Being a C-21 progestin, MPA has also glucocorticoid (22) and weak androgenic properties (8,31,39). MPA binds specifically and with a higher affinity than progesterone ($K_a = 1,3$ nM^{-1}) to the progesterone receptors in the human mammary tumor cytosol (69), but it has also been found to bind to the glucocorticoid receptor

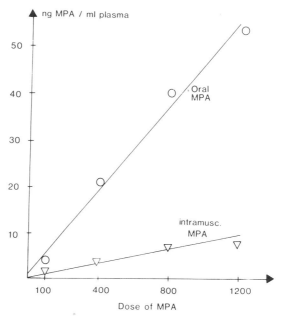

FIG. 1. Plasma concentrations of MPA 12 hr after oral and i.m. administration of single doses of MPA at dose levels ranging from 100 to 1200 mg.

in the mammary carcinomas (19,63) and to the androgen receptor in the rat prostate (31), and to the mouse kidney (39) and the human endometrium (33), albeit with low affinity for the latter two receptors. At the cellular level it is therefore conceivable that MPA given at high doses may affect mammary tumor growth by binding not only to the progesterone receptor, but also to the glucocorticoid and androgen receptors.

Even at high concentrations, progestins do not compete for binding to the estrogen receptor in the MCF-7 cell line (70) or in rodent uterus (5). The antagonistic action of progestins to estrogen action is of a noncompetitive nature in that progestins interfere with the replenishment of the ER molecules, which results in a decrease of the ER concentration in the target tissue (24,25,54).

PHARMACOLOGY

Various routes of administration have been used to elucidate the pharmacokinetics of MPA (9,23,59). After intravenous administration, a half-life of 4 hr has been reported (18,64). Following administration by the oral route, absorption of MPA takes place immediately. The highest blood levels are observed after 2–7 hr (13,59), and measurable amounts can be detected in the blood for several days or weeks, depending upon the dose (13,59). After intramuscular administration, the blood concentration of the drug increases slowly, reaching a peak after 2 days (13,59) and then decreases very slowly with an estimated half-life of 6 weeks (29). Following

TABLE 1. Overall treatment results

Author	Year	Ref.	No. of eval. pts.	PD[a] (No.)	NC[a] (No.)	PR (No.)	CR (No.)	CR+PR (No.)	%	95% CL%[b]
Andersen	1980	2	19	10	3	6	0	6	32	13–57
Castiglione and Cavalli	1980	10	9	NI	NI	6	0	6	32	13–57
De Lena et al.	1979	14	81	41	17	20	3	23	28	19–40
Goldberg	1968	19	108	NI	NI	—10—		10	9.2	5–17
Gorins et al.	1981	20	48	NI	NI	10	6	16	33	20–48
Izuo et al.	1981	28	20	6	7	7	0	7	35	15–59
Klaassen et al.	1976	30	40	NI	NI	—4—		4	10	3–24
Mattsson	1978	35	25	11	7	7	0	7	28	12–49
Mattsson	1980	36	26	5	7	9	5	14	54	33–73
Muggia et al.	1968	40	30	NI	NI	— 7—		7	23	10–42
Pannuti et al.	1980	44	168	51	41	73	3	76	45	37–53
Robustelli	1981	55	28	6	14	—8—		8	28	13–49
Robustelli et al.	1978	57	101	32	26	—43—		43	42.5	33–53
Salimtschik et al.	1980	60	31	20	6	3	2	5	16	5–34
Tominaga et al.	1981	67	49	NI	NI	11	3	14	28.5	17–43
Total no.				182/499	128/499			246/793		
Response (%)				36.4	25.6			31.0		
Range (%)				19–65	16–50			9–54		

[a]NI, not indicated.
[b]CL, confidence limits.

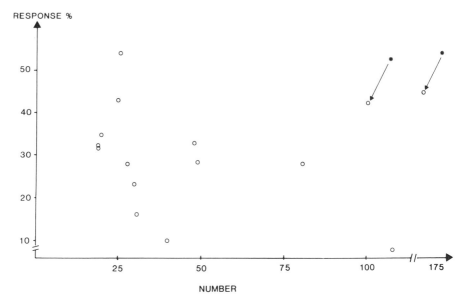

FIG. 2. Response rate in relation to number of evaluable patients in individual trial.

TABLE 2. *Response (CR + PR) in relation to dose and route of administration*

	Route of administration			
Dose level	Oral	Ref.	Intramuscular	Ref.
0–0.5 g	11/113 = 10%	2,19	12/49 = 39%	40,44,57
0.6–1.0 g	29/87 = 23%	2,60,67	81/222 = 36%	10,14,20, 35,36,57
> 1.0 g	28/76 = 37%	28,44,67	56/130 = 41%	14,44
Total	59/276 = 21%		183/477 = 38%	

daily oral or intramuscular administration of MPA the blood concentration reaches a steady state after 1–3 weeks (17,61).

The concentration of MPA in the plasma as a function of the dose and the route of administration is shown in Fig. 1 (59). It can be seen that the plasma concentration of MPA increases linearly with dose, regardless of whether the drug was administered orally or intramuscularly. Furthermore, it should be noted that the total dose exposure to MPA is the same for the two routes of administration over a given period of time (59).

The metabolic clearance rate for MPA (MCR[MPA]) is lower than the rate for progesterone, and as for other progestins there seems to be a large individual variation in the MCR[MPA] (21).

TABLE 3. *Response (PR + CR) in relation to dominant site of disease*

Author	Ref.	Soft tissue	Bone	Visc.
Castiglione and Cavalli	10	0/2	5/15	1/2
Goldberg	19	3/14	3/33	4/61
Klaasen et al.	30	1/7	0/17	1/16
Mattsson	35	0/1	2/3	5/21
Mattsson	36	0/1	2/7	12/18
Pannuti et al.	44	13/31	56/87	7/50
Robustelli et al.	57	6/20	25/46	12/35
Salimtschik et al.	60	4/18	0/3	1/10
Total		27/94	93/211	43/213
Response rate %		28.7	44.0	20.1

TABLE 4. *Side effects*

Abscess	64/443	14%
Infiltration	49/320	15%
Weight gain	65/107	61%
Moon face	34/238	14%
Vaginal bleeding	25/369	7%
Other	111/646	17%

PATIENT POPULATION

The clinical trials reviewed met the following criteria:

1. At least 15 evaluable female patients in the trial;
2. All patients treated with MPA;
3. Clear statements of criteria for response (compatible with those defined below);
4. Documentation of relevant data such as side effects, dominant site of disease, etc.

When reviewing the literature we found 42 papers dealing with MPA treatment of breast cancer. Among these one study has not been included in this review due to lack of definition of response criteria (62), another study because less than 15 patients were included in the trial (65). The lack of documentation of relevant data other than the remission rate led to the exclusion of three papers (7,11,12). Three papers were written in Italian with only a short English summary, which also led to exclusion from this review (1,4,41). Some authors included the same patient material in more than one paper. In these cases only the latest follow-up paper has been reviewed (43–53), although it has been necessary with regard to some aspects to go back to the previously published material.

One study has been excluded because both men and women entered the treatment (34). Furthermore, one study with adjuvant MPA treatment (42) and studies with MPA in combination with other systemic treatment (6,15,32,56) have not been included in this review and are only referred to in the discussion. Thus, 15 papers fulfilled the above-mentioned criteria for inclusion in this review.

CRITERIA OF RESPONSE

The major difficulty encountered in summarizing the experience with MPA in advanced breast cancer was the variety of criteria denoting response. However, except as stated, we have classified responses according to the following criteria:

1. Complete remission (CR): complete disappearance of all clinical disease;
2. Partial remission (PR): a more than 50% reduction in the size of some or all lesions, without concomitant increase of other lesions or appearance of new lesions;
3. No change (NC): a less than 50% reduction in the size of some or all lesions, without the appearance of new lesions or concomitant increase in other lesions of more than 25%;
4. Progressive disease (PD): a more than 25% increase in the size of any lesion(s) or the appearance of new lesions.

Some investigators did not distinguish between CR and PR (19,30,40,55,57). One author has classified the response in bone lesions as partial remission if the radiological findings were unchanged with simultaneous pain relief, thus using a mixture of objective and subjective criteria (44).

Another author (57) rated patients as being in remission if more than 50% of nonosseous lesions decreased in size, while all osseous lesions remained static, which may tend to give a too high response rate according to the UICC response criteria.

OVERALL TREATMENT RESULTS

Table 1 summarizes the overall results irrespective of previous systemic therapy and irrespective of dose and route of administration. In all, 793 patients are included in this review. The average rate of response to therapy was 31% with a range from 9 to 54%, and in a further 26% no change was achieved with a range from 16 to 50%.

The duration of response, including mean or median values, ranged from 20 to 58 weeks.

Figure 2 relates the response rate to the number of evaluable patients in the individual trial. As can be seen, there is a very wide range, but except in two studies (marked with an asterisk) it seems that the response rate decreases with an increasing number of patients in the trial, which emphasizes the importance of exercising caution in drawing conclusions from small studies. The two specially marked studies are those previously mentioned with differing response criteria (44,57).

RESPONSE TO MPA RELATED TO DOSE AND
ROUTE OF ADMINISTRATION

The response rate to MPA may depend on the dose level and the route of administration. In the papers reviewed MPA has been administered by two different routes, orally and intramuscularly. The results from studies employing different routes of administration and different dose levels of MPA are summarized in Table 2. As can be seen, the response rate seems to rise with increasing dose via the oral route, whereas the response rate with intramuscular administration does not seem to depend on the dose at the specific levels examined. The results in this table must be treated with extreme caution, as none of the patients within the three dose levels chosen were treated in randomized trials.

RESPONSE TO MPA RELATED TO DOMINANT SITE OF DISEASE

Eight papers presented sufficient information to allow for the analysis of this relation. As can be seen in Table 3, it seems that the highest response rate is achieved in bone lesions followed by soft tissue and viscera lesions. However, again it should be emphasized that one author (44), who observed very high response rates in bone lesions, classified pain relief and no objective change in bones as a partial remission.

RESPONSE TO MPA RELATED TO OTHER
PATIENT CHARACTERISTICS

Response to MPA related to disease-free interval and to steroid receptor content is not described in the papers dealt with. Similarly, rate of response related to menopausal age and previous systemic therapies was insufficiently described to allow for reasonable analyses.

SIDE EFFECTS

Eight of the papers reviewed have described the side effects of the treatment (Table 4). Abscesses and local infiltration occur in 14 and 15%, respectively, of the patients receiving MPA by the intramuscular administration. Among the other side effects it appears that many of these should be ascribed to the glucocorticoid action of MPA. Other side effects not listed in the table included acne, sweating, fine tremor, muscular cramps, hypertrichosis, nausea, and vomiting, hypercalcemia, constipation, thrombophlebitis, and water retention. Most of the side effects were rare, and generally all side effects were mild and did not require dosage modification. It should be emphasized, however, that although many of the symptoms are described as occurring during MPA treatment, they are not necessarily ascribable to this treatment. It is noteworthy that no evidence of hepatic disorders is described.

DISCUSSION

In spite of the extensive use of MPA over the last 20 years it is apparent that the present knowledge concerning the exact position of MPA in the treatment of advanced breast cancer is limited.

The average response rate is about 30%, and somewhat higher when the disease is localized mainly in soft tissue and bones, rather than in viscera. This tallies with the response rates of other endocrine treatment modalities. However, response rate related to previous systemic therapy and to important prognostic factors, such as age of the patients, disease-free interval, and hormone-receptor content of the tumor tissue, is only insufficiently elucidated. In view of the patient-to-patient variation in the metabolic clearance rate (21) data are still awaited from prospective randomized trials analyzing response rate in relation to dose and route of administration. One such trial comparing 300 mg/day to 900 mg/day, administered orally, is now in progress in the EORTC Breast Cancer Cooperative Group (16), as well as another randomized study in Denmark comparing oral with intramuscular treatment with MPA (3).

MPA has been used in combination with chemotherapy (6,32,56,68). In randomized trials some authors have reported varying degrees of additional effects (56,68), which could not be confirmed in other studies (6). Again, these conflicting results may be ascribed to different evaluation criteria, schedules of administration, and dosages. New prospective studies in these areas should be carried out once the optimal dosage has been defined.

In one study MPA was used as an adjuvant in comparison to radiotherapy (42). No difference was observed as regards the disease-free interval. Also in this respect, the efficacy of MPA should be reanalyzed once exact knowledge of dosage is available.

In view of the modest side effects of MPA treatment and the clinical and theoretical evidence of a mode of action different from that of other endocrine therapies, MPA is a drug with interesting qualities. Therefore, future controlled studies with MPA, both alone and in combination with other systemic therapies, should be performed in order to establish the position of MPA therapy in primary and advanced disease.

REFERENCES

1. Amadori, D., Ravaioli, A., and Barbanti, F. (1977): *Min. Med.*, 68:3967–3980.
2. Andersen, A. P. (1980): *MPA Symposium in Ulleåborg, Finland. (Personal communication)*.
3. Andersen, A. P., Brincker, H., Kjær, M., Frederiksen, P. L., Jakobsen, A., and Møller, K. Å. (1981): *Radium Center Århus, Odense and Herlev, Denmark*.
4. Bernardo-Strada, M. R., Imparato, E., Aspesi, G., Pavesi, L., and Robustelli Della Cuna, G. (1980): *Min. Med.*, 71:3241–3246.
5. Bonton, M. M., Martin, P. M., and Raynaud, J. P. (1979): *Cancer Treat. Rep.*, 63(7):1151.
6. Brunner, K. W., Sonntag, R. W., Alberto, P., Senn, H. J., Hartz, G., Obrecht, P., and Maurice, P. (1977): *Cancer*, 39:2923.
7. Bugalossi, P. (1963): *The Practitioner*, 191:702.
8. Bullock, L. P., Bardin, C. W., and Sherman, M. R. (1978): *Endocrinology*, 103:1768–1782.
9. Castegnaro, E., and Sala, G. (1971): *Steroidologia*, 2:13.
10. Castiglione, M., and Cavalli, F. (1980): *Schweiz. med. Wschr.*, 110:1073–1076.
11. Cooperative Breast Cancer Group (1961): *Cancer Chemother. Rep.*, 11:109–141.
12. Cooperative Breast Cancer Group (1964): *Cancer Chemother. Rep.*, 41:1–24.
13. Cornette, J. C., Kirton, K. T., and Duncan, G. W. (1971): *J. Clin. Endocrinol. Metab.*, 33:459–466.

14. De Lena, M., Brambilla, C., Valagussa, P., and Bonadonna, G. (1979): *Cancer Chemother. Pharmacol.*, 2:175–180.
15. Dogliotti, L., Mussa, A., and Di Carlo, F. (1979): *Cancer Treat. Rep., Abstr.*, 63:1219.
16. EORTC Breast Cancer Cooperative Group (1980): Protocol 10802.
17. Farlutal Review. *Farmitalia* (1977).
18. Fotherby, K., Kamyab, S., Littleton, P., and Klopper, A. (1965): *Endocrinology*, 33:XIII.
19. Goldberg, I. S. (1968): *Cancer*, 23:109–112.
20. Gorins, A., Gisselbrecht, C., Belpomme, D., Namer, M., and Juret, P. (1981): *Proc. XII International Congress Chem.*, Florence, Italy, no. 271.
21. Gupta, C., Osterman, J., Santen, R., and Bardin, C. W. (1979): *J. Clin. Endocrinol. Metab.*, 48:816–820.
22. Hellmann, L., Yoshida, K., Zumoff, B., Levin, J., Kream, J., and Fukushima, D. K. (1976): *J. Clin. Endocrinol. Metab.*, 42:912–917.
23. Helmrich, M. L., and Huseby, R. A. (1965): *Steroids*, 6:79–83.
24. Hsueh, A. J. W., Peck, Jr., E. J., and Clark, J. H. (1975): *Nature*, 254:337–339.
25. Hsueh, A. J. W., Peck, Jr., E. J., and Clark, J. H. (1976): *Endocrinology*, 98:438–444.
26. Huggins, C. (1965): *Cancer Res.*, 25:1163–1175.
27. Huggins, C., Moon, R. C., and Morrii, S. (1962): *Proc. Natl. Acad. Sci.*, 48:379–386.
28. Izuo, M., Iino, Y., and Endo, K. (1981): *Proc. XII International Chem.*, Florence, Italy, no. 273.
29. Jeppson, S., and Johansson, E. D. B. (1976): *Contraception*, 14:461–469.
30. Klaassen, D. J., Rapp, E. F., and Hirte, W. E. (1976): *Cancer Treat. Rep.*, 60:251–253.
31. Labrie, F., Drouin, J., Ferland, L., Lagace, L., Beaulieu, M., De Lean, A., Kelly, P. A., Caron, M. G., and Raymond, V. (1978): In: *Recent Progress in Hormone Research, Vol. 34*, edited by R. O. Greep, pp. 25–93. Academic Press, New York.
32. Longueville, J., and Maisin, H. (1975): *Adriamycin*, Parte IV:260–268.
33. Machaughlin, D. T., and Richardson, G. S. (1979): *J. Steroid Biochem.*, 10:371–377.
34. Madrigal, P. L., Alonso, A., Manga, G. P., and Modrego, S. P. (1980): In: *Role of Medroxyprogesterone in Endocrine-Related Tumors*, edited by S. Iacobelli and A. Di Marco, pp. 93–96. Raven Press, New York.
35. Mattsson, W. (1978): *Acta Radiol. Oncol.*, 17:387–400.
36. Mattsson, W. (1980): In: *Role of Medroxyprogesterone in Endocrine-Related Tumors*, edited by S. Iacobelli and A. Di Marco, pp. 65–71. Raven Press, New York.
37. McCormick, G. M., and Moon, R. C. (1973): *Europ. J. Cancer*, 9:483–486.
38. McGuire, W. L., Pearson, O. H., and Segaloff, A. (1975): In: *Estrogen Receptors in Human Breast Cancer*, edited by W. L. McGuire, P. P. Cargone, and E. P. Vollmer, p. 17. Raven Press, New York.
39. Mowszowicz, I., Bieber, D. E., Chung, K. W., Bullock, L. P., and Bardin, C. W. (1974): *Endocrinology*, 95:1589–1599.
40. Muggia, F. M., Cassileth, P. A., Ochoa, Jr., M., Flatow, F. A., Gellhorn, A., and Hyman, G. A. (1968): *Ann. Intern. Med.*, 68:328–337.
41. Mussa, A., Dogliotti, L., and Di Carlo, F. (1980): *Min. Med.*, 71:391–400.
42. Pannuti, F. (1978): *Arch. Geschwulstforsch.*, 48:680–682.
43. Pannuti, F. (1979): *Onkologie*, 2:54–60.
44. Pannuti, F., Di Marco, A. R., Martoni, A., Fruet, F., Strocchi, E., Burroni, P., Rossi, A. P., and Cricca, A. (1980): In: *Role of Medroxyprogesterone in Endocrine-Related Tumors*, edited by S. Iacobelli and A. Di Marco, pp. 73–92. Raven Press, New York.
45. Pannuti, F., Fruet, F., and Cricca, A. (1977): *IRCS Med. Sci.*, 5:433.
46. Pannuti, F., Martoni, A., Cricca, A., and Strocchi, I. (1977): *IRCS Med. Sci.*, 5:528.
47. Pannuti, F., Martoni, A., Di Marco, A. R., Piana, E., Saccani, F., Becchi, G., Mattiolo, G., Barbanti, F., Marra, G. A., Persiani, W., Cacciari, L., Spagnolo, F., Palenzona, D., and Rocchetta, G. (1979): *Europ. J. Cancer*, 15:593–601.
48. Pannuti, F., Martoni, A., Fruet, F., and Cricca, A. (1979): *Cancer Treat. Rep., Abstr.*, 63:1219.
49. Pannuti, F., Martoni, A., Fruet, F., Strocchi, E., and Di Marco, A. R. (1980): *Europ. J. Cancer*, Suppl. 1:93–98.
50. Pannuti, F., Martoni, A., Lenaz, G. R., Piana, E., and Nanni, P. (1978): *Cancer Treat. Rep.*, 62:499–504.
51. Pannuti, F., Martoni, A., and Piana, E. (1977): *IRCS Med. Sci.*, 5:54.

52. Pannuti, F., Martoni, A., Piana, E., and Fruet, F. (1977): *IRCS Med. Sci.*, 5:49.
53. Pannuti, F., Martoni, A., Pollutri, E., Camera, P., Losinno, F., and Giusti, H. (1976): *Pan. Med.*, 18:129–136.
54. Pavlik, E. J., and Coulson, P. B. (1976): *J. Steroid Biochem.*, 7:369–376.
55. Robustelli Della Cuna, G. (1981): *Proc. XII International Congress of Chemotherapy,* Florence, Italy, no. 384.
56. Robustelli Della Cuna, G., and Bernardo-Strada, M. R. (1980): In: *Role of Medroxyprogesterone in Endocrine-Related Tumors*, edited by S. Iacobelli and A. Di Marco, pp. 53–64. Raven Press, New York.
57. Robustelli Della Cuna, G., Calciati, A., Bernardo-Strada, M. R., Bumma, C., and Campio, L. (1978): *Tumori*, 64:143–149.
58. Sadoff, L., and Lusk, W. (1974): *Obstet. Gynecol.*, 43:262–266.
59. Salimtschik, M., Mourisden, H. T., Løber, J., and Johansson, E. (1980): *Cancer Chemother. Pharmacol.*, 4:267–269.
60. Salimtschik, M., Mouridsen, H. T., and Rose, C. (1980): *Unpublished data.*
61. Sall, S., DiSaia, P., Morrow, C. P., Mortel, R., Prem, K., Thigpen, T., and Creasman, W. (1979): *Am. J. Obstet. Gynecol.*, 135:647–650.
62. Segaloff, A., Cuningham, M., Rice, B. F., and Weeth, J. B. (1967): *Cancer*, 20:1673–1678.
63. Shyamala, G. (1974): *J. Biol. Chem.*, 249:2160–2163.
64. Slaunwhite, W. R., and Sandberg, A. A. (1961): *J. Clin. Endocrinol.*, 21:753–764.
65. Stoll, B. A. (1967): *Brit. Med. J.*, 3:338–341.
66. Stoll, B. A. (1967): *Cancer*, 20:1807–1813.
67. Tominaga, T., Izuo, M., Enomoto, K., Takatani, O., Kubo, K., and Nomura, Y. (1981): *Proc. XII International Congress of Chemotherapy*, Florence, Italy, no. 272.
68. Tucker, W. G., Stott, P. B., Zelkowitz, L., and Kubrika, M. (1974): *Proc. XI International Cancer Congress*, 3:600 *(Abstr.)*.
69. Young, P. C. M., Keen, F. K., Einhorn, L. H., Stanich, B. M., Ehrlich, C. E., and Cleary, R. E. (1980): *Am. J. Obstet. Gynecol.*, 137:284–292.
70. Zava, D. T., and McGuire, W. L. (1978): *Science*, 199:787–788.

*Role of Medroxyprogesterone in Endocrine-
Related Tumors, Volume II*, edited by L.
Campio, G. Robustelli Della Cuna, and R. W.
Taylor. Raven Press, New York © 1983.

Medroxyprogesterone Acetate High Dose and Bromocriptine: Results of a 4-Year Study in Stage IV Breast Cancer

Luigi Dogliotti, *Antonio Mussa, and **Francesco Di Carlo

*Clinica Medica B, *Clinica Chirurgica A, **Istituto di Farmacologia, University of
Turin, 10100 Turin, Italy*

The presence of specific receptor proteins for steroid hormones in about two-thirds of primary or metastatic breast cancers is well established. At present this biochemical marker represents the best available criterion for predicting the response of patients with advanced cancer to hormonal manipulations, and this is an excellent aid for anybody involved in treatment of breast cancer patients (17,24).

However, in addition to the better knowledge of the role of sexual hormones, evidence has been emerging that a mammotrophic pituitary hormone—prolactin (PRL)—could be involved in regulation of breast tumor growth, at least in a supportive role, not only in animal models (42,44) but also in humans (10,20, 23,27,31,33,42). Even though conflicting data are often reported on this matter, the recent detection of specific prolactin receptors (PRL-R) in about 35–50% of human breast cancer, with apparent lack of correlation with steroid receptors (4,5,15,32), indirectly supports the importance of this hormone as a growth factor in benign and malignant breast neoplasias. Underestimation of the possible influence of PRL in breast tumors could explain why the usual endocrine therapies are often disappointing, even in selected patients.

On the basis of these considerations we carried out a 4-year clinical trial in the management of patients with advanced breast cancer, selected or not selected for the "receptor status," with an original combination of two different drugs: medroxyprogesterone acetate (MPA-HD) and bromocriptine, a well-known semisynthetic ergot alkaloid, which is able to assure a significant and long-lasting decrease of PRL secretion. This trial began in 1976. Preliminary results have previously been reported (9,26).

MATERIALS AND METHODS

Between January 1976 and January 1980, 70 patients with well-documented advanced breast cancer entered this trial. Patients were considered eligible for inclusion in our study if they had measurable tumor parameters that could be followed when looking for a response to therapy. Patients with the presence of central nervous system lesions were excluded. All 70 patients were evaluable. The main characteristics of patients are summarized in Table 1.

All patients were naturally menopausal or had previously undergone surgical oophorectomy. About 80% of patients were submitted to our therapy as a first step therapy; the remaining had previously received chemotherapy or X-ray therapy. In all cases disease was clearly progressive.

The pretreatment and follow-up examinations included full clinical assessment, serum biochemistry, chest and skeletal X-ray, isotope bone, liver, and brain scan and, as required, echography and computerized tomography (CT). In some cases with suspected liver involvement, a liver biopsy, through laparascopy, was also done.

Metastases were placed, in order of frequency, in skin, soft tissues, bones, lung, and liver. Many patients had two or more sites involved, with a very poor Karnofsky index. In all patients plasma prolactin and gonadotropins [luteinizing hormone (LH); follicle-stimulating hormone (FSH)] concentration was measured between 8 and 9 A.M. by a sensitive double antibody radioimmunoassay (RIA kit, Sorin, Saluggia; Italy). In the meantime plasma cortisol concentration was measured by a competitive protein binding assay. In some patients plasma dehydroepiandrosterone sulfate (DHA-S) values were also assessed. The hormonal evaluations were carried out at least three times before treatment, and repeated every 10 days during the first month of therapy; subsequently evaluations were done every 3 months until relapse.

Forty-seven out of seventy patients were submitted to the research and quantitative analysis of estradiol (ER) and progesterone (PgR) receptors in primary or metastatic localizations, with dextran-coated charcoal assay (DCC) and Scatchard-plot analysis (3); binding capacity was expressed as femtomoles (10^{-15} Mol) per mg of cytosol protein.

Thirty-seven out of forty-seven patients were considered receptor-positive (R+) for the presence of ER and/or PgR in neoplastic tissue, at concentrations more than

TABLE 1. *Main characteristics of patients*

Total patients	70
Median age	54 (range: 32–78)
Free interval (months)	
median	36
range	0–240
Dominant site of metastases	
soft tissue	23 (33%)
osseous	31 (45%)
visceral	16 (22%)
Steroid receptor	
>5 fmol/mg cytosol protein (R+)	37 (54%)
<5 fmol/mg cytosol protein (R−)	10 (14%)
not determined	23 (32%)

5 femtomoles/mg cytosol protein; 10 patients were considered receptor-negative
(R −). In the remaining 23 patients treated, it was not possible to obtain information
about the "receptor status" (R not determined).

All patients entering the trial were placed on MPA 1 g/day × 30 days, then 1
g every 5 days i.m.; meanwhile bromocriptine was given orally 2.5 mg four times
a day (Table 2). If positive results were achieved, this treatment was not discontinued
until progression of the disease was evinced.

All patients were hospitalized during the initial 10 days of treatment; then they
were usually followed as outpatients by us. Strict emphasis was placed on punctual
observance of the dose and the time of administration of drugs scheduled.

The criteria for assessment of patient response were in accordance with those
recommended by UICC (12). Complete remission (CR) is considered to be the
disappearance of all lesions, with recalcification of lytic bone metastases. Partial
remission (PR) is a 50% decrease in measurable lesions, without appearance of
new lesions. No change (NC) is recorded when the lesions, on the whole, are
unchanged, even if subjective improvement occurred. Progression (P) is recorded
when some or all lesions progress or new lesions appear, as well as when some
lesions regress while others progress.

Only CR and PR were considered positive results, but NC patients also continued
to receive MPA + bromocriptine until progression. Progressive patients and those
who progressed after a positive or no change response, were crossed to polichemotherapy (FAC/CMF) + MPA at lower dosage. The duration of remission is recorded from the day when the patients started the therapy.

RESULTS

Overall objective results are shown in Table 3. Thirty-eight patients (54%) had
a positive result; twenty-three (33%) showed a complete response. Clear progression
occurred in twenty-one (30%).

Objective responses according to dominant site are showed in Table 4. Responding patients with bone metastases, many of them with massive involvement of
skeleton, severe pain, and walking impairment, showed a dramatic relief of pain
after a few days of treatment and progressive improvement of walking in the
subsequent days. An unexpected 69% of positive responses were recorded in visceral
lesions, many of them being liver metastases, as pointed out by liver biochemistry,
repeated scanning, echography, CT, and subjective improvement.

Table 5 shows responses according to "receptor status." There was no significant
difference in overall positive responses in R+ patients compared to R-not-deter-

TABLE 2. *MPA-HD and bromocriptine:*
Schedule of treatment

MPA	1 g/day × 30 days i.m.
	then 1 g every 5 days i.m.
Bromocriptine	2.5 mg × 4/day × os

TABLE 3. *MPA-HD + bromocriptine:*
Overall objective response

Response[a]	Patients (N = 70)[b]	
CR	23 (33)	38 (54)
PR	15 (21)	
NC	11 (16)	
P	21 (30)	

[a]CR, complete remission; PR, partial remission; NC, no change; P, progression.
[b]Numbers in parentheses represent percentages of patients treated.

TABLE 4. *MPA-HD + bromocriptine: Overall objective response*
according to dominant site

	CR	PR	NC	P
Soft tissue (N = 23)	7 (30)	1 (4)	6 (20)	9 (39)
Osseous (N = 31)	10 (32)	9 (29)	5 (16)	7 (22)
Visceral (N = 16)	6 (38)	5 (31)	—	5 (31)

CR, complete remission; PR, partial remission; NC, no change; P, progression. Numbers in parentheses represent percentages of patients tested.

TABLE 5. *MPA-HD + bromocriptine: Objective response according*
to "receptor status"

Response[a]	R+ (N = 37)		R− (N = 10)		R not det. (N = 23)	
CR	16 (43)	(59)	2 (20)	(30)	5 (22)	(57)
PR	6 (16)		1 (10)		8 (35)	
NC	8 (22)		1 (10)		2 (8)	
P	7 (19)		6 (60)		8 (35)	

Numbers in parentheses represent percentages of patients treated.
[a]CR, complete remission; PR, partial remission; NC, no change; P, progression.

mined patients (59 versus 57%). Nevertheless it is noteworthy that R+ patients showed progressive disease only in 19% of cases, while progression occurred in 35% of R not determined patients. Moreover CR occurred in 43% of R+ patients in comparison with 22% of R not determined patients. These data appear impressive, but statistical analysis shows only a trend to be significant ($p = 0.1$, Fischer exact test), possibly because the high disparity in the initial number of treated patients. R− patients showed only 3 positive responses out of 10 patients treated.

The actuarial life-table analysis of duration of response in overall responding patients (CR + PR + NC)—as determined by Kaplan–Meyer survival curves for nonparametric observations (18)—shows a median duration of response at 24 months (range 8–48 + months). About 50% of patients are still responding after 4 years of observation (Fig. 1).

Shown in Fig. 2 is the persistence of remissions of patients who achieved a positive response (CR + PR). Stratification was done between patients R + and patients R not determined. In the first group (22 patients) median is not reached at 44 months, while in the second (13 patients) median was reached at 21 months of observation. Of 3 patients with negative steroid receptor who achieved a positive response, one had a recurrence after 8 months of treatment, the others recurred between 12 and 15 months of observation.

HORMONE DATA

As shown in Figs. 3 and 4 mean plasma PRL, FSH, LH, and cortisol values were in the normal range for menopausal women before treatment. During the first 2 weeks of treatment all the hormonal values tested decreased in a significant manner. Then these low values were maintained during all the length of treatment. In particular (Fig. 3) PRL levels fell from 18 ± 3 ng/ml (mean $\pm$ SEM) to 2 ± 1 ng/ml and cortisol from 15 ± 3 µg%ml to 2 ± 1 µg%ml. In some cases plasma cortisol was undetectable. FSH decreased from 90 ± 21 to 27 ± 13 mU/ml and LH from 75 ± 15 to 9 ± 2 mU/ml. All the differences observed were statistically highly significant ($p < 0.01$).

Regarding the behavior of hormonal values, no differences were observed between responding and nonresponding patients. Concerning androgens derived from the adrenals studied by plasma DHA-S changes, actuarial data are not sufficient for statistical evaluation, because of the great variance of basal levels. Nevertheless in most patients studied, we saw a clear-cut trend to lowering of DHA-S levels, with values similar to those recently reported in advanced breast cancer by Santen et al. (39) with aminogluthetimide plus hydrocortisone.

DRUG SIDE EFFECTS

Principal side effects are summarized in Table 6. Bromocriptine side-effects occurred in the initial stages of treatment: gastric pain, nausea, and vomiting were the most common. To minimize these symptoms we usually started with a lower dose of the drug (1.25 mg twice a day), taken with meals, gradually increasing 2.5 mg every 2 days. No patients showed hemorrhagic gastritis nor peptic ulcera. In some patients dryness of mouth, leg cramps, and hyperkinesis also occurred. Four patients suffered from acute orthostatic hypotension in the first day of treatment: this symptom disappeared promptly and did not appear again throughout treatment duration.

During the first month of therapy with high daily doses of MPA, glutea abscess occurred in about 8% of patients; nevertheless we were never obliged to discontinue the therapy. In the following months of treatment glutea abscess decreased to 1–2% of patients; in some cases we stopped parenteral administration, crossing to oral administration, 100 mg four times a day. After 10–12 months of therapy

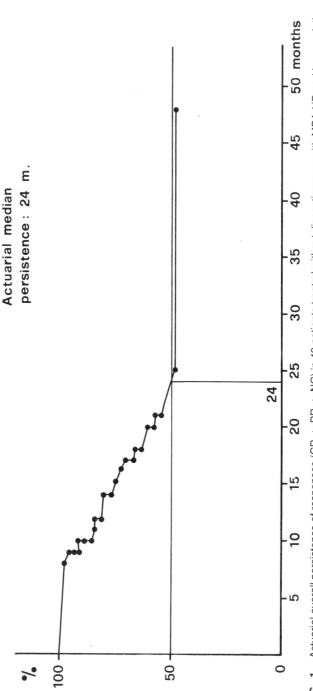

Actuarial median persistence : 24 m.

FIG. 1. Actuarial overall persistence of responses (CR + PR + NC) in 49 patients treated without discontinuance with MPA-HD and bromocriptine.

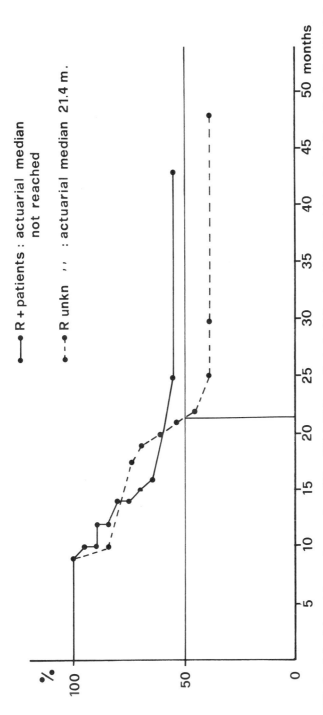

FIG. 2. Actuarial persistence of regressions (CR + PR) in 22 R + patients *(solid lines)* and in 13 R-not-determined patients *(broken lines)* treated without discontinuance with MPA-HD and bromocriptine.

R + patients : actuarial median not reached

R unkn ,, : actuarial median 21.4 m.

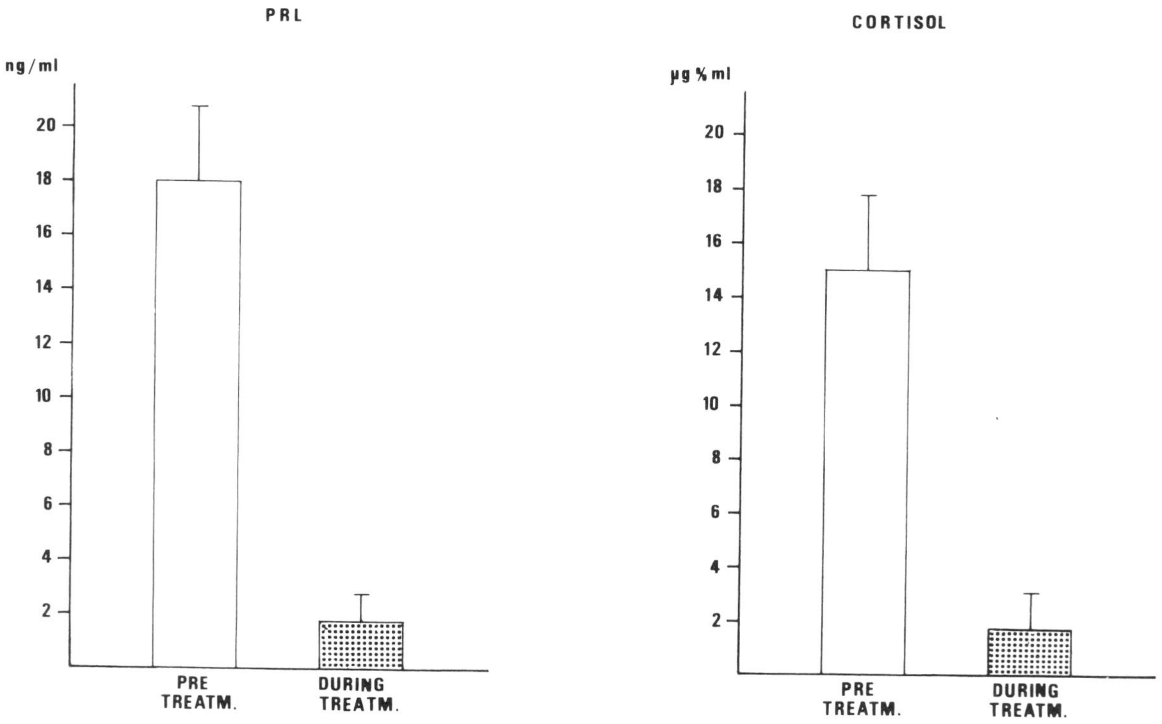

FIG. 3. PRL and cortisol plasma basal values (mean ± SEM) before and during treatment with MPA-HD and bromocriptine.

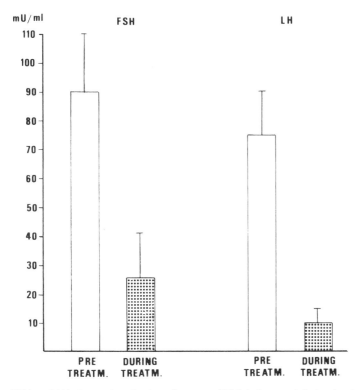

FIG. 4. FSH and LH plasma basal values (mean ± SEM) before and during treatment with MPA-HD and bromocriptine.

TABLE 6. *MPA-HD bromocriptine: Main side effects*

Bromocriptine	Gastric pain, nausea, and vomiting in the beginning of therapy
	Orthostatic hypotension in 4 patients
MPA	8% glutea abscess in the first month of therapy
	Moderate Cushing-like effect in 40%
	Systolic hypertension in 20%

moderate Cushing-like effects occurred in 40% of patients. Systolic arterial pressure increased significantly in 20% of patients; vaginal spotting in 10%. After 1 or 2 years of therapy a group of patients were randomly allocated to receive endometrial biopsy: endometrial histological modifications were never observed.

No significant changes in common hematological tests were observed, except for 2 patients who showed moderate hyperglicemia. Both in the beginning of treatment and after years of treatment, thrombopnlebitis events or cardiac pathology were never evinced. On the whole, side effects were always of slight consequence, never obliging us to discontinue the scheduled treatment.

DISCUSSION

The reevaluation of endocrine therapy in the management of breast cancer during these last years has been largely dependent on the new biochemical understanding of the action of hormones in normal and neoplastic breast tissues. New drugs, generally acting as "antihormones," such as tamoxifen, aminogluthetimide, and MPA high doses, are actually in trial, in order to obtain, as much as possible, positive results with the lowest side effects and to spare major ablative surgery, like adrenalectomy or hypophysectomy.

The combined use of high doses of MPA and bromocriptine in management of stage IV breast cancer in menopausal women, was done in order to obtain a selective medical hypophysectomy with direct peripheral antiestrogenic effect. The rationale for this therapy is outlined in Fig. 5. Strong reduction of pituitary gonadotropin production by MPA is well documented (35,38) and confirmed by our data. Moreover large doses of MPA lower cortisol production rate and plasma cortisol values by a negative feedback action on the hypothalamus or pituitary (13); also adrenal androgen production, and thereby extraovery estrogen source, is lowered by MPA (11). So a real "medical adrenalectomy" occurs. This finding appears to be very important, considering the recent evidence of the active conversion of adrenal estrogen precursors in estrone, particularly by the malignant breast tissue (34). Besides being MPA free of estrogenic properties, it does not show any prolactin-stimulating effect (28) and could probably depress the hypoglicemic release of growth hormone (41).

It has been well known for some time that progesterone is able to antagonize or modify the action of estrogens at their target tissues. However, it has only recently been shown that the mechanism by which progesterone affects the action of estradiol on the uterus is related to a reduction in the synthesis of cytoplasmic ER (16). Di Carlo et al. (3) showed that MPA high doses *in vivo* decrease the binding capacity of estradiol to its specific uterine receptors and confirmed *in vitro* its ability to interfere with the binding of estradiol to cytosol receptors obtained from human estrogen-dependent breast tumor (6,7). Moreover, the same authors showed that MPA-HD reduces the synthesis of cytoplasmic ER (Fig. 6).

It is extremely likely that, in comparison with those obtained in the past, the more favorable results recently reported in breast and uterine cancer by several investigators, using MPA at high doses (1,2,22,29,30,37) are largely dependent on this directly inhibiting effect of progestins on the number and binding activity of ER.

Bromocriptine is a long-acting dopaminergic drug which suppresses PRL secretion activating dopaminergic inhibitory PRL control mechanism at the hypothalamus and hypophyseal level (43). This drug is actually the best to be employed for PRL suppression; long-term therapy with daily doses of 7.5–10 mg results in continued suppression of PRL for the entire day. Our data not only confirmed this finding but showed that PRL suppression is maintained during years of treatment, providing that the drug is never stopped.

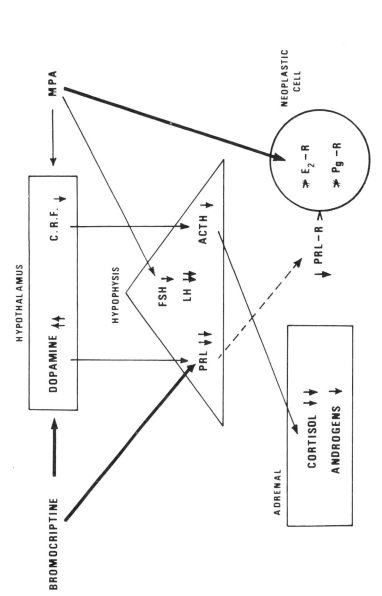

FIG. 5. Scheme of MPA and bromocriptine main effects on the hypothalamus–hypophysis–adrenal axis and on neoplastic breast cell.

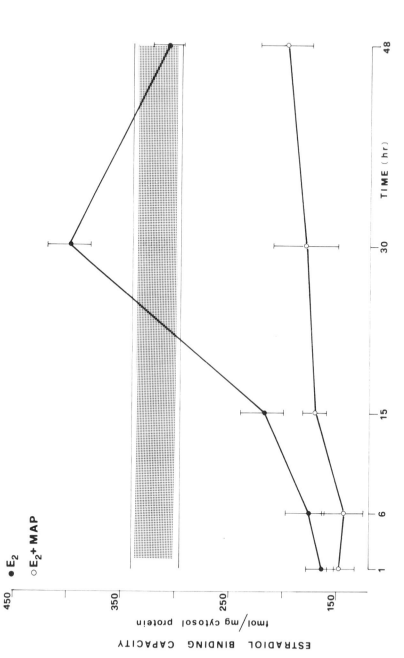

FIG. 6. Effect of administration of 10 ng i.p. estradiol 17β alone (*solid circles*) or with MPA (*open circles*) (20 mg/kg orally), given 5 min later, on the binding of (^{3}H)-estradiol-17β to its specific uterine cytosolic receptors in the rat. Results are means ± SEM of four determinations with 20 rats in each group. *Shaded area*, range of basal values (untreated animals).

Bromocriptine, as well as a similar PRL-suppressing drug, lergotrile, employed as single drug in management of patients with advanced breast cancer, gave discouraging results (14,32,40). However, all patients treated were unselected for possible hormonodependence.

The presence of PRL receptors in 35–50% of breast cancer (4,5,32), the possible interrelationship between PRL-R and sexual steroids (19) and between bromocriptine and ER (5), and finally the proved usefulness of bromocriptine in the management of benign breast lesions (8,21,25) show that this topic needs more investigation.

The administration of massive doses of MPA combined with bromocriptine induced a positive response in 54% of overall treated patients. In patients selected for the presence of steroid receptors, 59% positive results were obtained; in unselected patients, 57%. Three patients out of ten treated with negative receptors responded well.

Because our study has to be considered as a "pilot study," without randomization of patients, only historical comparison can be made. The overall acute responses appear to be similar or somewhat better to those reported for tamoxifen or aminogluthetimide in comparable patients, and better with regard to MPA-HD alone.

Striking differences appear in the number of CR versus PR, particularly in R + patients. Moreover liver metastases, usually not responding at all or responding poorly to hormonal manipulations, showed a very satisfactory number of good responses.

Our results corroborate the importance of receptor determinations in predicting response to therapy, in particular for R − patients. However the good results also obtained in unselected patients, in term of acute responses and persistence of responses, make this combined treatment likely to represent a good first approach in unselected advanced breast cancer.

The most interesting data to come from our investigation are the excellent results obtained in persistence of responses. The approximately 50% of overall patients still in remission after 4 years' therapy and the more than 50%, only considering R + patients, is an unforeseen result. Certainly, continuing the treatment until clear progression, when acute positive results are achieved, is probably the most important reason why the results achieved are so much better in comparison with intermittent therapy. Besides, it is possible to speculate that this combined therapy, interfering with the synthesis or the peripheral action of a number of hormones involved in breast cancer growth, is able to cause, within the months of therapy, a natural selection of patients: the ones with a prevalence of cellular clones containing steroid and/or PRL receptors continue to respond to hormonal therapy, the others cease to respond after a shorter time.

In conclusion, MPA-HD appears to be a satisfying and well-tolerated therapy in women with stage IV breast cancer: possible associations—combined or sequential—appear interesting, particularly chemohormonotherapy (36). With respect to combined progestins–anti-PRL therapy, some results we obtained appear impressive. Obviously they should be confirmed with randomized trials. A more accurate stratification of patients, at least as regards our proposed therapy, should be fulfilled when prolactin receptors will also be involved. This is the aim of our next trial, which is now in progress.

ACKNOWLEDGMENTS

This work was supported in part by a grant of Consiglio Nazionale delle Ricerche (CNR), Special Project "Control of Neoplastic Growth," contract n°80.01598.96. Authors are indebted to Dr. Sergio Sandrucci, Clinica Chirurgica A, for skillful assistance in patients' management and to Dr. Fulvio Agrimonti, Clinica Medica B, for statistical analysis of the study.

REFERENCES

1. Bonte, J., Decoster, J. M., Ide, P., and Billet, G. (1978): *Gynecol. Oncol.*, 6:70–75.
2. De Lena, M., Brambilla, C., Valagussa, P., and Bonadonna, G. (1979): *Cancer Chemother. Pharmacol.*, 2:175–180.
3. Di Carlo, F., Conti, G., and Reboani, C. (1978): *J. Endocrinol.*, 77:49–55.
4. Di Carlo, R., and Muccioli, G. (1979): *Tumori*, 65:695–702.
5. Di Carlo, R., Muccioli, G., Conti, C., Reboani, C., and Di Carlo, F. (1980): In: *Pharmacological Modulation of Steroid Action*, edited by E. Genazzani, F. Di Carlo, and W. I. P. Mainwaring, pp. 261–266. Raven Press, New York.
6. Di Carlo, F., Pacilio, G., and Conti, G. (1975): *Tumori*, 61:501–508.
7. Di Carlo, F., Reboani, C., Conti, G., Portaleone, P., Viano, I., and Genazzani, E. (1980): In: *Pharmacological Modulation of Steroid Action*, edited by E. Genazzani, F. Di Carlo, and W. I. P. Mainwaring, pp. 261–746. Raven Press, New York.
8. Dogliotti, L., and Mussa, A. (1981): *J. Endocrinol. Invest.*, 4 *(suppl. 1)*, 433–435.
9. Dogliotti, L., Mussa, A., and Di Carlo, F. (1978): In: *Current Chemotherapy, Vol. II*, edited by W. Siegenthaler and R. Luthy, pp. 1287–1289. American Society for Microbiology, Washington.
10. Friesen, H. G. (1976): In: *Breast Cancer: A Multidisciplinary Approach*, edited by G. St-Arneault, P. Band, and L. Israel, pp. 143–149. Springer-Verlag, Berlin, Heidelberg, New York.
11. Grattarola, R. (1976): *J. Natl. Cancer Inst.*, 56:11–16.
12. Hayward, J. L., Carbone, P. P., Heuson, J. C., Kumaoka, S., Segaloff, A., and Rubens, R. D. (1977): *Europ. J. Cancer*, 13:89–94.
13. Hellman, L., Yoshida, K., Zumoff, B., Levin, J., Kream, J., and Fukushima, D. K. (1976): *J. Clin. Endocrinol. Metab.*, 42:912–917.
14. Heuson, J. C., Coume, A., and Staquet, M. (1972): *Europ. J. Cancer*, 8:155–156.
15. Holdaway, I. M., and Friesen, H. G. (1977): *Cancer Res.*, 37:1946–1952.
16. Hsueh, A. J. W., Peck, E. J., and Clark, J. H. (1976): *Endocrinology*, 98:438–444.
17. Iacobelli, S., King, R. J. B., Lindner, H. R., and Lippman, M. E., editors (1980): *Hormones and Cancer*. Raven Press, New York. `
18. Kaplan, E. L., and Meyer, P. (1958): *J. Am. Statist. Assoc.*, 53:457–481.
19. Kelly, P. A., Djiane, J., and De Léan, A. (1980): In: *Central and Peripheral Regulation of Prolactin Function*, edited by R. M. McLeod and U. Scapagnini, pp. 173–188. Raven Press, New York.
20. Leung, C. K. H., and Shiu, R. P. C. (1981): *Cancer Res.*, 41:546–551.
21. Mansel, R. E. (1981): *Research and Clinical Forums*, 3:61–65.
22. Mattsson, W. (1978): *Acta Radiol. Oncol.*, 17:387–400.
23. McGuire, W. L. (1977): In: *Prolactin and Human Reproduction*, edited by P. G. Crosignani and C. Robyn, pp. 143–151. Academic Press, London, New York, San Francisco.
24. McGuire, W. L., Horwitz, K. B., Zava, D. T., Garola, R. E., and Chamness, G. C. (1978): *Metabolism*, 27:487–501.
25. Mussa, A., and Dogliotti, L. (1979): *J. Endocrinol. Invest.*, 2:87–89.
26. Mussa, A., Dogliotti, L., and Di Carlo, F. (1980): *Min. Medica*, 71:391–400.
27. Nagasawa, H. (1979): *Europ. J. Cancer*, 15:267–279.

28. Namer, M., Krebs, B., Lupo, R., Cambon, P., Abbes, M., and Lalanne, C. M. (1976): In: *Hormones and Breast Cancer*, edited by M. Namer and C. M. Lalanne, pp. 181–192. INSERM, Paris.
29. Pannuti, F., Di Marco, A. R., Martoni, A., Fruet, F., Strocchi, E., Burroni, P., Rossi, A. P., and Cricca, A. (1980): In: *Role of Medroxyprogesterone in Endocrine-Related Tumors*, edited by S. Iacobelli, A. Di Marco, pp. 73–92. Raven Press, New York.
30. Pannuti, F., Martoni, A., Lenaz, G. R., Piana, E., and Nanni, P. (1978): *Can. Treat. Rep.*, 62:499–504.
31. Pearson, O. H., Arafah, B., and Manni, A. (1980): In: *Central and Peripheral Regulation of Prolactin Function*, edited by R. M. McLeod and U. Scapagnini, pp. 237–242. Raven Press, New York.
32. Pearson, O. H., and Manni, A. (1978): In: *Current Topics in Experimental Endocrinology, Vol. III*, edited by L. Martini and V. H. T. James, pp. 75–92. Academic Press, London, New York.
33. Pearson, O. H., Manni, A., Chambers, M., Brodkey, J., and Marshall, J. S. (1978): *Cancer Res.*, 38:4323–4326.
34. Perel, E., Wilkins, D., and Killinger, D. W. (1980): *J. Steroid Biochem.*, 13:89–94.
35. Pérez-Palacios, G., Fernandez-Aparicio, M. A., Medina, M., Zacarias-Villareal, J., and Ulloa-Aguirre, A. (1981): *Acta Endocrinol.*, 97:320–328.
36. Robustelli della Cuna, G., and Bernardo-Strada, M. R. (1980): In: *Role of Medroxyprogesterone in Endocrine-Related Tumors*, edited by S. Iacobelli and A. Di Marco, pp. 53–64. Raven Press, New York.
37. Robustelli della Cuna, G., Calciati, A., Bernardo-Strada, M. R., Bumma, C., and Campio, L. (1978): *Tumori*, 64:143–149.
38. Sadoff, L., and Lusk, W. (1974): *Obstet. Gynecol.*, 43:262–267.
39. Santen, R. J., Worgul, T. J., Samojlik, E., Interrante, A., Boucher, A. E., Lipton, A., Harvey, H. A., White, D. S., Smart, E., Cox, C., and Wells, S. A. (1981): *New Engl. J. Med.*, 305:545–551.
40. Schultz, K. D., Czygan, P. J., Del Pozo, E., and Friesen, H. G. (1973): In: *Human Prolactin*, edited by J. P. Pasteels and C. Robyn, pp. 268–276. Excerpta Medica, Amsterdam.
41. Simon, S., Schiffer, M., Glick, S. M., and Schwartz, E. (1967): *J. Clin. Endocrinol. Metab.*, 27:1633–1636.
42. Smithline, F., Sherman, L., and Kolodny, M. D. (1975): *New Engl. J. Med.*, 15:784–789.
43. Thorner, M. O., Fluckiger, E., and Calne, D. B., editors (1980): *Bromocriptine. A Clinical and Pharmacological Review*. Raven Press, New York.
44. Welsch, C. W., and Nagasawa, H. (1977): *Cancer Res.*, 37:951–963.

Role of Medroxyprogesterone in Endocrine-Related Tumors, Volume II, edited by L. Campio, G. Robustelli Della Cuna, and R. W. Taylor. Raven Press, New York © 1983.

Concurrent Hormonal and Cytotoxic Treatment for Advanced Breast Cancer

G. Robustelli Della Cuna, Q. Cuzzoni, P. Preti, and G. Bernardo

Division of Oncology, Clinica del Lavoro Foundation, University of Pavia, 27100 Pavia, Italy

Since the survival of women with disseminated breast cancer has not improved greatly in recent years, the current goal of medical treatment still remains to achieve the longest survival in the greatest number of patients. In the past, disseminated disease has been initially treated with hormonal therapy, while single-drug chemotherapy was assigned to patients who failed to respond to one or more endocrine manipulations. Afterwards the use of multidrug chemotherapy instead of single-drug treatment significantly improved the response rate and survival of women with metastatic disease, challenging the traditional position of endocrine treatment as first line therapy of advanced breast cancer (31,38,40).

Subsequently the possibility of determining cytosol steroid receptors in primary and metastatic breast cancer tissues (10,17,18) revalued the role of endocrine therapy in a large subset of patients. Notwithstanding the high percentage of response achieved with both cytotoxic (4) and endocrine treatments (25), the survival of women with clear evidence of tumor regression has plateaued at 18–24 months, in contrast to 8–10 months for those not responding (12,40). The obvious shortcomings of either above-mentioned therapeutic modalities are the low incidence of complete responses (until now in the range of 8–20%), together with the short duration of response and survival. Nowadays, like 10 years ago, there is an urgent need to overcome this critical situation. The choice of treatments capable of improving results lies between two possibilities: the search of new active agents or the combination of singly active modalities. Apart from the discovery of new effective drugs, the attempts to combine chemotherapy and immunotherapy were disappointing (1). At the moment chemo- and hormonotherapy is one of the therapeutic means from which a further improvement of results is expected. Empirically started in the seventies (13,14), combined endocrine and cytotoxic therapy has been subsequently rationalized on the basis of new emerging knowledge on breast cancer biological characteristics (steroid receptors content, hormone-specific receptor interactions, heterogeneous nature of the cell population of human breast cancer) (31,35). At the same time experimental (8,34) and clinical data (2,5,7,11,12,21,31) supported the validity of this approach. Nevertheless, although many clinical experiences are in favor of combined chemo- and hormonal treatment, the results so far obtained in disseminated breast carcinoma are equivocal (2,5,11,31–33).

CHEMO- AND HORMONOTHERAPY REVISITED

Since the data of controlled clinical trials are not many (23,25), only the results obtained in randomized prospective studies will be considered here. Ablative procedures have been combined with cytotoxic therapy both in pre- and postmenopausal women with advanced breast cancer (2,7,21,24). The Swiss Group for Clinical Cancer Research (SAKK), demonstrated that in premenopausal patients with receptor status unknown, oophorectomy plus multidrug chemotherapy is superior to chemotherapy alone (2); the response with combined treatment was 74% with a median duration of response of 9.5 months and a median survival of 19.9 months. By itself cytotoxic therapy obtained 43% response rate with a median duration of 7.8 months and survival of 13.2 months. Even if not statistically significant, the differences suggests a trend in favor of combined approach. These results were later confirmed by the experience published by Falkson et al. (7) on behalf of Cancer and Leukemia Group B (CALGB). One hundred and fifty-seven premenopausal women with metastatic carcinoma of the breast were prospectively randomized to receive either ovariectomy followed by observation until progression, or ovariectomy plus single-agent chemotherapy (cyclophosphamide), or ovariectomy plus combined chemotherapy (cyclophosphamide/methotrexate/fluorouracil/vincristine/prednisone). The complete plus partial response rates were 18, 65, and 72%, respectively. While the percentage response following oophorectomy plus either single-agent or combined chemotherapy were significantly better than that observed with ovariectomy alone, the differences in survival among the three treatment arms failed to reach statistical significance. However, the results of the CALGB trial suggest a clear advantage of concurrent chemo- and hormonotherapy as compared with ovariectomy alone.

In postmenopausal patients the data regarding ablative procedures are few and generally not conclusive (11). In this group of patients additive hormonotherapy with various compounds (estrogens, androgens, low-dose progestins, and corticosteroids) has been combined with different chemotherapeutic regimens (31,37). Diethylstilbestrol given concurrently with single or multidrug chemotherapy seems to increase response rate, median duration of response and, sometimes, survival in postmenopausal unselected women with disseminated disease. Androgens, combined with single or multiple cytotoxic agents chemotherapy, have hitherto given conflicting results. Testolactone and nandrolone decanoate plus single-drug chemotherapy failed to obtain better results than chemotherapy alone. The weakly androgenic calusterone in combination with cyclophosphamide/fluorouracil/prednisone (CFP) gave the same response rate as did CFP alone; conversely, when used concurrently with adriamycin and cyclophosphamide (AC), calusterone gave a significantly higher response rate and longer duration of response and survival (12,31). In a study by the Eastern Cooperative Oncology Group (ECOG), specifically designed to evaluate the impact of chemo- and hormonotherapy upon maintenance of response in advanced breast cancer, the androgen fluoxymesterone (added to cyclophosphamide/methotrexate/fluorouracil combination) showed its ability to increase the median time to progression (38). After 6 months' induction with three cytotoxic regimens (adriamycin/vincristine), CMF (cyclophosphamide/methotrexate/fluorouracil), and CMF plus prednisone, the benefit from adding fluoxymesterone was pronounced only in partial responders. In this subset of patients the addition of fluoxymesterone increased the time to failure from 5.3 to 10.8 months. Low-dose progestins (medroxyprogesterone acetate less than 500 mg/i.m./day, norethisterone acetate 20–30 mg/day/orally) have been added to chemotherapy without any beneficial effect either in response rate or in survival (2,31,33). A clear evidence of objective tumor regression from corticosteroids alone is infrequent and, wh n it occurs, is generally of short duration. Prednisone by itself gives only a limited number of responses in metastatic breast cancer (35). Notwithstanding in some prospective clinical trials (9) it proved its capacity to enhance the effectiveness of two cytotoxic combinations CMFV (cyclophosphamide/methotrexate/flourouracil/vincristine) and CMF, at least in terms of increased response rate. Conversely, when added to adriamycin-containing regimens, prednisone did not improve results (9). Until now the role of prednisone in the chemohormonal therapy of disseminated breast cancer is not clearly defined and further studies are needed to clarify available conflicting results.

NEW AGENTS FOR CONCURRENT CHEMOHORMONOTHERAPY

Among agents thought most suitable for combination with chemotherapy, the antiestrogen tamoxifen (TMX) and high-dose medroxyprogesterone acetate (HD-MPA) deserve special attention. TMX, a synthetic nonsteroidal compound with a potent antiestrogenic activity, has a structure very similar to diethylstilbestrol. It has been used mainly in unselected postmenopausal women bearing metastatic disease with overall results ranging between 22 and 38% (19). Even though higher response rate to concurrent TMX and polichemotherapy, as compared with chemotherapy alone, have been reported (Table 1), there are data yet incomplete and there are conflicting opinions on its real capacity to prolong survival in women with disseminated disease (5,11,31,32,37).

As a single agent medroxyprogesterone acetate (MPA), a synthetic steroid derived from progesterone, until 1973 has given poor results in advanced breast cancer (31). With low doses (40–400 mg/day) overall response rate did not exceed 20% for a median duration of no more than 6 months. Starting from 1974 the position of MPA was revised and it has since been considered an effective agent in the management of metastatic breast cancer (30). This change of attitude hinged upon the use of high doses (≥500 mg/day/i.m.) of HD-MPA. A couple of prospective controlled clinical trials (22,29) demonstrated that the optimun parenteral dose of this compound is 500 mg/day for 30 days, as induction, followed by the same dose twice a week as maintenance therapy. The indications derived from clinical experiences have recently been confirmed by pharmacokinetic data (36).

TABLE 1. *Clinical results of tamoxifen plus polychemotherapy in postmenopausal women with advanced breast cancer*

Author(s)	Ref.	Regimen[a]	No. of pts.	Response rate (%)	Survival (median/mos.)
Robustelli, Della Cuna et al. (1979)	31	TMX		26	—
		TMX + LMFVP	196	46	—
		TMX→LMFVP		51	—
Tormey (1980)	37	DA	28	38	—
		TMX + DA	33	64	—
Cocconi et al. (1981)	5	CMF	71	51	29.5
		TMX + CMF	62	74	21.0
Rosso et al. (1981)	32	CMF	20	40	Not yet reached
		TMX + CMF	20	75	at 24 mos.

[a]L, chlorambucil; M, methotrexate; F, fluorouracil; V, vincristine; P, prednisone; C, cyclophosphamide; D, dibromodulcitol; A, adriamycin; TMX, tamoxifen; (+) concurrent, (→) delayed.

TABLE 2. *Clinical results of MPA plus polychemotherapy in postmenopausal women with advanced breast cancer*

Authors	Ref.	Regimen	No. of pts.	Response rate (%)	Survival (median/mos.)
Brunner et al. (1977)	2	CMFVP	37	63	22.8
		MPA+CMFVP[a]	38	53	18.1
Pellegrini et al. (1980)	23	CAMF	24	45	21.5
		MPA + CAMF	21	61	28.0
Robustelli, Della Cuna et al. (1980)	28	FAC	40	55	16
		MPA + FAC	40	75	28

[a]MPA = low-dose medroxyprogesterone acetate. For other abbreviations see footnote of table 1.

Together with TMX, HD-MPA may be considered at the moment as one of the most effective hormonal compound in the treatment of disseminated breast cancer (19,25,26,28,29,31). This statement remains valid even though some recently published papers (6,15) suggest a more cautious interpretation of the previously reported results (more than 40% response rate and median duration of response of 10 months). The explanation of different opinions on that topic lies probably in the characteristics of the treated patients. In fact, in early trials only previously untreated patients were admitted, whereas the most recent controlled studies included only heavily pretreated women with advanced mammary carcinoma, who had become resistant to previous chemotherapy and/or endocrine treatment. In our opinion it is just in this kind of patient that HD-MPA demonstrates its therapeutic activity as an effective agent capable of yielding response rates still ranging from 28 to 35%.

Combined treatment of HD-MPA and various chemotherapy regimens has been employed in advanced breast cancer with encouraging results (Table 2). In a three-arms prospective controlled study (28), 120 mostly previously untreated patients

with metastatic disease were randomized to receive (a) fluorouracil/adriamycin/
cyclophosphamide (FAC), (b) FAC plus HD-MPA i.m. and (c) FAC plus HD-MPA
orally. After a follow-up period of 48 months the results are those shown in Table
3. The concurrent use of parenteral HD-MPA and polychemotherapy gave a higher
response rate and median duration of responders survival significantly longer (29.5
months) that in the group treated by chemotherapy alone (18.5 months).

In a randomized trial Pellegrini et al. (23) compared the multidrug regimen CAMF
(cyclophosphamide/adriamycin/methotrexate/fluorouracil) with the same plus HD-
MPA orally in 50 patients with disseminated breast cancer. Chemotherapy alone
gave 45.8% of responses; median duration, 10.9 months; overall median duration
of survival, 21.5 months as compared with 61.9% response rate; median duration
of response, 22.5 months; overall median duration of survival, 28.5 months of
chemo- and hormonotherapy group. At 5 years from the start of treatment responders
still alive were 9% on CAMF and 23% in CAMF plus HD-MPA groups, respectively. As chemohormonal treatment including HD-MPA is concerned, two interesting aspects have to be considered. The first relates to the dose of MPA, which
must also be high ($\geq$500 mg/day) when concurrently administered with chemotherapy. It has been shown in fact that the daily dose of MPA is a critical factor
(15,22,25,31). Moreover it seems that some reported therapeutic failure (2) of
chemo- and hormonotherapy containing MPA could be ascribed to the use of low
dose of this progestin. The second interesting finding is that, in combination with
cytotoxic agents, HD-MPA is more active than TMX in causing improvement of
performance status, pain relief, feeling of well being, and in protecting bone marrow. Marrow toxicity induced by prolonged use of cytotoxic agents seems actually
less in the HD-MPA-treated groups of patients in both previous mentioned studies
(23,28). Although nobody knows what this really means, the above cited "protective" effect of MPA on bone marrow has been already described for prednisone,

TABLE 3. *Four-year results of HD-MPA plus polychemotherapy in advanced
breast cancer*

	FAC alone	FAC + MPA (500 mg/im.)	FAC + MPA (500 mg/orally)
Overall response rate (CR + PR)[a]	55	75	65
Median duration of response (months)	9[b]	19[b]	13
Overall median survival (months)	16	28	22
Median responders survival	20[c]	31.5[c]	24
Still alive			
overall	4/40 (10%)	9/40 (22%)	5/40 (12.5%)
responders	2/22 (9%)	7/30 (23%)	4/26 (15%)

[a]CR, complete response; PR, partial response.
[b]$p < .001$
[c]$p < .05$ (log-rank test).

fluoxymesterone, and norethisterone, when concurrently used with chemotherapy (9,33,37,38). The ability of these hormones to bolster bone marrow reserve would seem to permit the administration of higher doses of myelotoxic drugs. On the basis of these observations it could be argued that the superior results obtained by combining endocrine therapy with cytotoxic drugs might be ascribed only to so-called protective effect of hormones on bone marrow, which would allow a more strictly adhered to treatment schedule. In our experience (28), even if a trend in favor of the two MPA-treated groups of patients seems to exist, the calculation of the total average percentage of the administered doses did not show any statistically significant difference between each arm of the study (Table 4). Furthermore both experimental (20) and clinical observations (39) really support the concept of a direct cytotoxic effect of MPA, which, acting in a synergistic way with chemotherapy, could actually explain the encouraging results so far reported (23,28).

CONCLUSIONS AND OUTLOOKS

In advanced breast cancer, irrespective of some exciting but never subsequently confirmed results (3,16), a further improvement of response rate and survival is unlikely to be obtained with traditional chemotherapy or hormonal treatment. Moreover experimental and laboratory data give a good rationale for a combined chemo and hormonal approach (8,27,34). It seems likely that by adding estrogens, androgens, corticosteroids, antiestrogens, and high doses of MPA to polychemotherapy we can achieve better results than with chemotherapy alone (31). Notwithstanding the above-mentioned results, it does not mean that the concurrent use of hormones and cytotoxic drugs is superior to other possible combinations (i.e., intermittent or sequential). Until now, however, the attempts made (21,24) and ongoing experiences (11) of sequential chemohormonotherapy have failed to give conclusive results. Since guidelines on how to use at best hormonal manipulations and cytotoxic drugs are at present lacking, we have to remember what is well known and consequently to try to follow the best way to obtain the best results. Nowadays some of the following facts can be considered well established:

TABLE 4. *Average percentage of the optimal scheduled dose of polychemotherapy administered in each of the first eight cycles*

	Cycles[a]								Total average %
Regimen	1	2	3	4	5	6	7	8	
FAC alone	98	90	88	84	79	78	81	79	84.6
	(40)	(39)	(37)	(31)	(29)	(19)	(18)	(18)	
FAC + MPA i.m.	96	95	94	91	89	88	88	86	90.8
	(40)	(40)	(39)	(36)	(28)	(24)	(22)	(22)	
FAC + MPA orally	97	90	88	89	90	84	81	80	87.3
	(40)	(40)	(38)	(29)	(26)	(24)	(20)	(20)	

[a]Parentheses contain number of patients. For other abbreviations see footnotes of Table 2.

1. Adriamycin-containing regimens are superior to other combinations either in response rate and duration of response and survival (4,12). However, it is well recognized that adriamycin cardiotoxicity limits the possibility of using this drug for long periods of time. Otherwise it is widely accepted that low-dose adriamycin combinations produce worse results than full-dose programs. A possibility for by-passing this situation could be in maintaining the adriamycin dose within the range of 20–40 mg/m^2 for one cycle in every four in the attempt to reach the cumulative dose responsible for cardiotoxicity as late as possible. Since previously reported experience (12) gave encouraging results, two multicentric controlled clinical trials (see Appendix) are ongoing in order to evaluate the therapeutic efficacy of adriamycin/cyclophosphamide (AC) plus HD-MPA and vincristine/adriamycin/cyclophosphamide (VAC) plus HD-MPA as compared with the same chemotherapies alone in advanced breast cancer. Both trials have been designed with the aim of administering the antracycline derivative for as long as possible by saving adriamycin at each cycle (AC) or by delaying the time necessary to reach the total cumulative dose (VAC).

2. In postmenopausal women with disseminated disease TMX and HD-MPA seem the two most suitable compounds for combination with effective cytotoxic regimens. MPA, by virtue of previously described characteristics (23,28,31), seems to have more possibilities of giving better results than TMX in combined treatments (5,23,28).

Considering the extremely variable behavior of the disease in patients with breast cancer relapsed after primary treatment, chemo- and hormonal treatment at the moment cannot be considered the treatment of choice for every women with disseminated mammary carcinoma. Its real value should yet be tested, taking into account prognostic and risk factors as well as the steroid receptor characteristics of individual patients. Only by the identification of the subset of women eligible for treatment (27) will it be possible to clarify the impact of this combined approach on the course of the disease. Notwithstanding the encouraging successes so far obtained, the doubt still remains that whatever is gained initially as increased response rate and prolonged time to progression could be lost later in terms of survival. Such doubt is expected to be removed in the near future if the results of the ongoing clinical trials provide enough evidence that chemo- and hormonal combinations have been able to consistently prolong (beyond the limit of 3 years) the median survival time of the greatest number of women with metastatic breast carcinoma.

APPENDIX

A. Chemo- and hormonotherapy of advanced breast cancer: vincristine/adriamycin/cyclophosphamide (VAC) versus VAC plus high-dose medroxyprogesterone acetate (MPA).

Protocol CHEM-OR-MA 1/79 of Collaborating International Group for the Study of Breast Carcinoma. Coordinators: A. Pellegrini, G. Robustelli Della Cuna, and C. Praga.

Objectives: 1. Comparison of response rate, duration of response, and survival between chemotherapy and chemotherapy plus MPA; 2. Evaluation of changes on duration of survival with maintenance without adriamycin when a complete or partial response has been obtained; 3. Evaluation of the protective effects of MPA on bone marrow toxicity of chemotherapy.

Study design: Postmenopausal patients with progressive breast cancer, after stratification according performance status, previous therapy, and dominant site of lesions, are randomized to:

VAC→VCF→VACM→VCMF or to the same chemotherapeutic sequence plus high dose MPA.

Regimens: Patients, after randomization are treated in sequence (induction, consolidation, maintenance) with the following cycles: (a) Vincristine (V) 1 mg/i.v. day 1, adriamycin (A) 50 mg/m^2/i.v. day 1, cytoxan (C) 100 mg/m^2/orally days 1–8 every 21 days. (b) VFC where fluorouracil (F) 750 mg/m^2 i.v. day 1 replaces adriamycin, every 28 days. (c) VACM, here methotrexate is added to VAC regimen at the moment of progression. MPA is given at the daily dose of 500 mg/day i.m. for 2 weeks and then twice a week without discontinuity.

Progress: Since April 1981, 231 patients have been entered, the accrual of new cases was stopped in June 1981.

B. Comparative study of adriamycin/cyclophosphamide (AC) versus AC plus medroxyprogesterone acetate (MPA) in advanced breast cancer.

Protocol 182/81 of International Cooperative Study on Advanced Breast Cancer (Chairman: L. Campio).

Objectives: To determine the efficacy of MPA added to chemotherapy in comparison to chemotherapy alone in the treatment of advanced breast cancer.

Study design: Postmenopausal patients with progressive metastic disease stratified according performance status, free interval, and dominant site are randomized to chemotherapy or chemotherapy plus MPA.

Regimens: (a) Adriamycin 40 mg/m^2/i.v. on day 1, cyclophosphamide 200 mg/m^2 orally on days 3–6. The first three courses of AC administered at 3-week intervals and subsequently every 4 weeks. (b) Chemotherapy as above plus MPA 500 mg/i.m. × 28 days and then 500 mg orally until progression.

Progress: The trial is ongoing and the accrual of patients will be closed in June 1982.

REFERENCES

1. Blumenschein, G. R., Hortobagyi, G. N., Richman, S. P., Gutterman, J. U., Tashima, C. K., Buzdar, A. U, Burgess, M. A., Livingston, R. B., and Hersh, E. M. (1980): *Cancer*, 45:742–749.
2. Brunner, K. W., Sonntag, R. W., Alberto, P., Senn, H. J., Martz, G., Obrecht, P., and Maurice, P. (1977): *Cancer*, 39:2923–2933.
3. Bull, J. M., Tormey, D. C., Li, S. H., Carbone, P. P., Falkson, G., Blom, J., Perlin, E., and Simon, R. (1978): *Cancer*, 41:1649–1657.
4. Carbone, P. P., Bauer, M., Band, P., and Tormey, D. (1977): *Cancer*, 39:2916–2933.
5. Cocconi, G., De Lisi, V., Boni, C., Magnani, P., and Bertusi, M. (1981): *Proc. 12th International Congress of Chemotherapy*, Florence, Italy, Abstr. 383.

6. De Lena, M., Brambilla, C., Valagussa, P., and Bonadonna, G. (1979): *Cancer Chemother. Pharmacol.*, 0:175–180.
7. Falkson, G., Falkson, H. C., Glidewell, O., Weinberg, V., Leone, L., and Holland, J. F. (1979): *Cancer*, 43:2215–2222.
8. Formelli, F., Zaccheo, T., Casazza, A. M., Bellini, O., and Di Marco, A. (1981): *Europ. J. Cancer (in press)*.
9. Geimer, N. F., and Donegan, W. L. (1980): *Reviews on Endocrine-Related Cancer*, 6:5–11.
10. Jensen, E. V., De Sombre, E. R., and Jungblut, P. W. (1967): In: *Endogenous Factors Influencing Host-Tumor Balance*, edited by R. W. Wissler, T. L. Dao, and S. Wood, Jr., p. 15. University of Chicago Press, Chicago.
11. Jungi, W. F., Brunner, K. W., and Cavalli, F. (1980): *Reviews on Endocrine-Related Cancer*, 5 *(Suppl.)*, 29–42.
12. Lloyd, R. E., Jones, S. E., and Salmon, S. E. (1979): *Cancer*, 43:60–65.
13. Mannes, P., Derriks, R., and Moens, R. (1972): *Lille Med.*, 17:762–764.
14. Mannes, P., Derriks, R., Moens, R., Laurent, C., and Dalcq, J. M. (1976): *Cancer Treat. Rep.*, 60:85–89.
15. Mattson, W. (1978): *Acta Radiol. Oncol.*, 17:387–400.
16. Mattsson, W., Arwidi, A., Von Eyben, F., and Lindholm, C. E. (1977): *Cancer Treat. Rep.*, 61:1527–1531.
17. McGuire, W. L., Carbone, P. P., and Wollmer, E. P. editors (1975): *Estrogen Receptors in Human Breast Cancer*. Raven Press, New York.
18. McGuire, W. L., Raynaud, J. P., and Baulieu, E. E., editors (1977): *Progesterone Receptors in Normal and Neoplastic Tissue*. Raven Press, New York.
19. Mouridsen, H., Palshof, T., Patterson, T., and Battersby, L. (1968): *Cancer Treat. Rev.*, 5:131–141.
20. Natoli, C., Sica, G., and Iacobelli, S. (1981): *Tumori*, 67:185 (Abstr. 233).
21. Nemoto, T., Rosner, D., Diaz, R., Dao, T., Sponzo, R., Cunningham, T., Horton, J., and Simon, R. (1978): *Cancer*, 41:2073–2077.
22. Pannuti, F., Martoni, A., Di Marco, A. R., Piana, E., Saccani, F., Becchi, G., Mattioli, G., Barbanti, F., Morra, G. A., Persiani, W., Cacciari, L., Spagnolo, F., Palenzona, D., and Rocchetta, G. (1979): *Europ. J. Cancer*, 15:593–601.
23. Pellegrini, A., Massidda, B., Mascia, V., Pasqualucci, S., Desogus, A., and Monni, A. (1980): *Tumori*, 66 (Suppl.), 99 (Abs. 103).
24. Priestman, T., Baum, M., Jones, V., and Forbes, J. (1978): *Brit. Med. J.*, 2:1673–1674.
25. Robustelli Della Cuna, G. (1980): *Med. Biol. Environ.*, 8:371–377.
26. Robustelli Della Cuna, G. (1981): *Proceedings 12th International Congress of Chemotherapy*, Florence, Italy, Abstr. 384.
27. Robustelli Della Cuna, G. (1982): In: *Role of Tamoxifen in Breast Cancer*, edited by M. Lippman, S. Iacobelli, G. Robustelli Della Cuna, pp. 53–59. Raven Press, New York.
28. Robustelli Della Cuna, G., and Bernardo-Strada, M. R. (1980): In: *Role of Medroxyprogesterone Acetate in Endocrine-Related Tumors*, edited by S. Iacobelli and A. Di Marco, pp. 53–64. Raven Press, New York.
29. Robustelli Della Cuna, G., Calciati, A., Bernardo-Strada, M. R., Bumma, C., and Campio, L. (1978): *Tumori*, 64:143–149.
30. Robustelli Della Cuna, G., Imparato, E., and Bernardo, G. (1981): *Med. Biol. Environ.*, 9:527–534.
31. Robustelli Della Cuna, G., Pellegrini, A., and Ganzina, F. (1980): *Chemotherapy and Hormonal Treatment of Advanced Breast Cancer*. Farmitalia Carlo Erba Publisher, Milano.
32. Rosso, R., Boccardo, A., Rubagotti, A., and Guarneri, D. (1981): *Proceedings 12th International Congress of Chemotherapy*, Florence, Italy. Abstr. 385.
33. Rubens, R. D., Begent, R. H. J., Knight, R. K., Sexton, S. A., and Hayward, J. L. (1978): *Cancer*, 42:1680–1686.
34. Sluyser, M. (1979): *Biochem. Biophys. Acta*, 560:509–529.
35. Stoll, B. A. (1979): *Reviews on Endocrine-Related Cancer*, 1:29–37.
36. Tamassia, V., Battaglia, A., Ganzina, F., Isetta, A. M., Sacchetti, G., Cavalli, F., Goldhirsch, A., Brunner, K., Bernardo, G., and Robustelli Della Cuna, G. (1982): *Cancer Chemother. Pharmacol.*, 8:151–156.
37. Tormey, D. C. (1980): *Review on Endocrine-Related Cancer*, 4 *(Suppl.)*, 33–38.
38. Tormey, D., Gelman, R., Band, P., and Falkson, G. (1979): *Proc. Am. Soc. Clin. Oncol.*, 20:356.

39. Vecchietti, G., Gerzeli, G., Zanoio, L., Novelli, G. G., and Barni, S. (1979): *Min. Ginecol.*, 31:1–7.
40. Young, R. C., Lippman, M., De Vita, V. T., Bull, J., and Tormey, D. (1977): *Ann. Intern. Med.*, 86:784–798.

Role of Medroxyprogesterone in Endocrine-Related Tumors, Volume II, edited by L. Campio, G. Robustelli Della Cuna, and R. W. Taylor. Raven Press, New York © 1983.

Hormone Dependency and Hormone Responsiveness of Endometrial Adenocarcinoma to Estrogens, Progestogens, and Antiestrogens

J. Bonte

Gynecologic Cancerology, St. Rafaël Hospital, B-3000 Louvain, Belgium

Estrogens as such can be considered as co-carcinogens in relation to the origin of half of primary endometrial adenocarcinomas and to the appearance of their metastases and recurrences. These are hormone-dependent adenocarcinomas as opposed to the other so-called autonomous tumors, induced by nonhormonal as yet undetermined carcinogens.

The hormone dependency of some endometrial adenocarcinomas is evidenced by the convergence of some data we were able to collect. Approximately 70% of our postmenopausal patients present with an estrogenic vaginal smear (Table 1) (30). The hormone-dependent endometrial adenocarcinomas seem to be the more differentiated ones, characterized by pseudostratification and a high mitotic index, whereas the autonomous tumors are the less differentiated types, appearing in patients with an atrophic vaginal smear (Table 2). The presence of estrogens, mostly of extraovarian origin, in normal cyclical serum concentrations as well as in low postmenopausal concentrations could be sufficient to induce hormonal carcinogenesis. The serum estradiol concentrations are in the menopausal range (<0.11 mmol/liter) in approximately 65% of stage I endometrial carcinoma patients and in more than

TABLE 1. *Disseminated or recurrent uterine adenocarcinoma[a]*

Type of vaginal cytology	Patients (%)
Estrogenic	68
Intermediate	16
Atrophic	16

[a]115 postmenopausal (hyster-) ovariectomized patients treated by means of 1 gr MPA/week; preliminary hormonal evaluation of the host by vaginal cytology.

TABLE 2. *Relationship: Differentiation of endometrial adenocarcinoma to cytohormonal evaluation of vaginal smear*

Vaginal smear	Endometrial adenocarcinoma	
	differentiated (%)	undifferentiated (%)
Estrogenic	76	48
	$P < 0.01$	
Subatrophic or atrophic	24	52

80% of those with advanced or recurrent cancers; the values are on the same level for the hormone-dependent and the autonomous group. Even so, the serum estrone concentrations are in the menopausal range (<19 mmol/liter) in approximately 65% of stage I endometrial adenocarcinoma patients and in more than 80% of those with advanced or recurrent cancers; the values are on the same level for the hormone-dependent and the autonomous group (Fig. 1).

All these data seem to circumscribe the possible carcinogenicity of the estrogens as a simple qualitatively related mechanism rather than as a quantitatively related one.

This mechanism of action is confirmed by the *in vitro* study of the behavior of endometrial adenocarcinoma grown in organotypic culture, permitting the addition of steroid hormones to the medium. In that way was proved not only the direct mechanism of action of estrogens at the cellular level of the endometrial adenocarcinoma, but even the mitogenic, possibly carcinogenic activity of estradiol at physiologic normal cyclical or low menopausal concentrations on the endometrial adenocarcinoma. Thus, the causal influence of estrogens in the genesis of hormone-dependent endometrial adenocarcinomas is determined by the abnormal characteristics of the endometrium cell.

The importance of the cellular factor in the genesis under estrogenic stimulation of hormonal dependent endometrial adenocarcinomas seems evidenced by the phenomena of enhanced dedifferentiation and mitotic activity, increased incorporation of tritiated thymidine, and finally, depressed secretory activity, as they appear in endometrial adenocarcinomas grown in organotypic culture after addition of estradiol to the medium.

The hypothesis seems acceptable that the cellular target for the carcinogenic action of the estrogens should be the cytoplasmic, and perhaps the nuclear steroid receptors, especially the estrogen and progestogen receptors.

Some of our data seem to corroborate this hypothetic mechanism of action on estrogen-induced and, thus, hormone-dependent, endometrial adenocarcinomas. Cytosolic estrogen receptor levels are highest in differentiated, thus hormone-dependent tumors, and lowest in undifferentiated, mostly autonomous adenocarcinomas. The estrogenic appearance of the vaginal smear coincides with a lower level of estrogenic receptors in differentiated tumors, possibly either because some cytosol

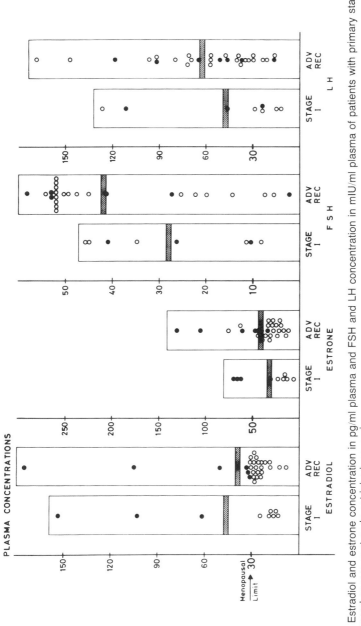

FIG. 1. Estradiol and estrone concentration in pg/ml plasma and FSH and LH concentration in mIU/ml plasma of patients with primary stage I or with advanced or recurrent endometrial adenocarcinoma.

receptor sites occupied by endogenous estrogens were not measured or because a fraction of the receptors had been transferred to the nuclei by the endogenous hormone or a combination of both possibilities (Fig. 2).

The estrogen and progestogen receptors could be presumed responsible for the regulation of the mitotic and secretory activity of the endometrium cell. Moreover, an abnormal receptor pattern could be at the origin of hyperplastic or even neoplastic degeneration of the endometrium. In that way, well or moderately differentiated hormone dependent endometrial adenocarcinomas should be characterized by the presence either of both cytosolic receptors with a lower than normal progestogen receptor/estrogen receptor ratio or of the estrogen receptor alone; autonomous, generally poorly differentiated adenocarcinomas on the contrary should either contain a very low estrogen receptor concentration or be devoid of both progestogen receptor and estrogen receptor.

In our experience, approximately 50% of endometrial adenocarcinomas are hormone dependent and could therefore, from a practical therapeutic viewpoint, be considered as hormone responsive to antiestrogenic drugs, progestogens, and antiestrogens (Table 3) (42–44).

The action of progestogens and antiestrogens on the endometrial adenocarcinoma presents a certain analogy including some identical phenomena together with many

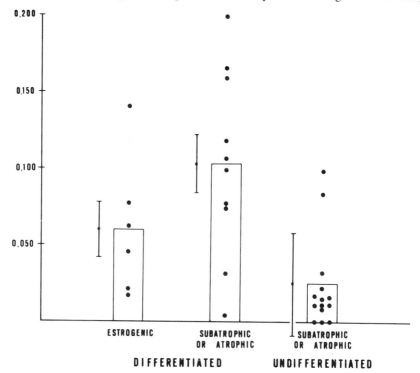

FIG. 2. Cytosolic estradiol receptor binding capacity in pmol/mg protein of endometrial adenocarcinoma in relationship to differentiation and cytohormonal evaluation.

TABLE 3. *Disseminated or recurrent uterine adenocarcinoma[a]*

Group	Cases treated	Responsiveness (%)
Responsive	58	51
Nonresponsive	57	49

[a]115 cases treated by means of 1 gr medroxyprogesterone/ week. Hormone dependency and responsiveness illustrated.

completely different mechanisms. In that way, a definite group of adenocarcinomas is equally sensitive to both drugs, while other types respond better either to progestogens or to antiestrogens.

RESPONSE OF ENDOMETRIAL ADENOCARCINOMA TO PROGESTOGENS

Progestogens neutralize the cytosolic estrogen receptor system in the endometrial adenocarcinoma cells, inhibiting the incorporation of tritiated thymidine, and thus the mitotic activity, and stimulating the various secretory activities. The histological response is characterized by:

the transformation of pseudostratified cells to active monolayered glands;
marked epithelial metaplasia of the glandular structures, especially in adeno-
    acanthomatous tumors;
pseudodecidualization of the stroma;
atrophy of the epithelium and fibrosis of the stroma, leading to the breakdown
    of the tumor substance.

Addition of progestogens to the medium of endometrial adenocarcinomas in organotypic culture reproduces the same histological transformations as described *in vivo* for the treated patients. These data show that progestogens attack the carcinoma locally by a direct mechanism of action at a cellular level (3,46).

The absence of statistically significant changes in steroid hormone plasma levels under high-dose medroxyprogesterone acetate (MPA) administration renders an indirect mechansim for action of progestogens on endometrial adenocarcinoma rather improbable. Indeed, administration of 1 g MPA per week induces no significant changes in estradiol and estrone plasma concentrations. The fall in follicle-stimulating hormone (FSH) plasma concentration during MPA treatment is statistically significant for the whole patient group; the fall of luteinizing hormone (LH) is only statistically significant for the responsive group (20).

After MPA treatment progestogen responsiveness is characterized by a sudden change towards atrophy in the vaginal smear, another hormonal target analogous to the endometrial adenocarcinoma (Table 4). In all hormone-dependent endometrial adenocarcinomas, administration of progestogens induces a rapid and significant

TABLE 4. *Disseminated or recurrent uterine adenocarcinoma[a]*

Vaginal cytohormonal response		Significant remission rate (%)
Estrogenic→	atrophic	
Estrogenic→	intermediate	96
Intermediate→	atrophic	
Estrogenic ⎫		
Intermediate ⎬	unchanged	11
Atrophic ⎭		
Mean reference rate		51

[a]115 postmenopausal (hyster-) ovariectomized patients treated by means of 1 gr medroxyprogesterone/week; predictive value of vaginal cytohormonal response to progestational treatment.

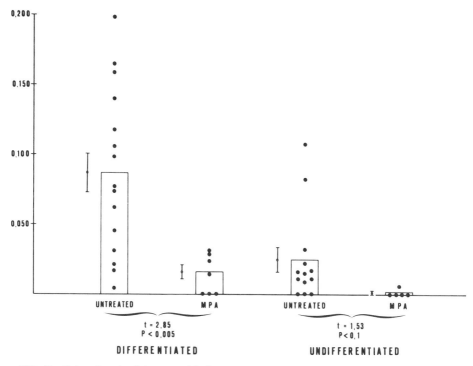

FIG. 3. Cytosolic estradiol receptor binding capacity in pmol/mg protein of primary or recurrent endometrial adenocarcinoma in relationship to differentiation and MPA treatment.

fall of estrogen receptor levels (Fig. 3) (29); cytosolic PR levels seems to be reduced by progestogen treatment (Fig. 4).

Evaluation of the therapeutic efficiency of progestogens either alone or as an adjuvant is based on clinical data.

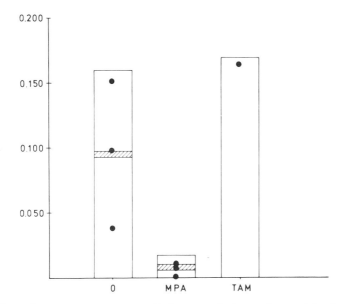

FIG. 4. Cytosolic progesterone receptor binding capacity in pmol/mg protein of primary or recurrent endometrial adenocarcinoma under MPA or tamoxifen treatment.

Hormone Therapy

In approximately 60% of the patients in our series with *in situ* endometrial carcinoma treated with progestogens, no residual cancer could be detected. The same oral or parenteral administration of progestogens in invasive stage I endometrial carcinoma completely destroyed the tumor in no more than 20% of the cases (17,21).

Local intracavitary application of progestogens was more effective in the eradication of invasive stage I endometrial carcinoma. After intrauterine instillation of progestogens, the tumor completely disappeared in approximately 35% of the cases. Intrauterine insertion of an MPA-releasing device achieved total destruction of malignant tissue in 60% of uteri which had no myometrial invasion (Table 5) (27).

Since the first publication by Kelley and Baker (33) on the treatment of advanced or recurrent uterine carcinoma with progestogens, at least 84 reports have provided data on responses to 11 different progestogens and analyzed the remission rate in about 3700 patients. Using the mean objective remission rate calculated per individual report, there is a difference between the responses to the various progestogens: 47% with MPA and 28% with 17-α-hydroxyprogesterone (17α-OHPC) (11,14).

In our most recent analysis of a series of 115 patients with advanced or recurrent endometrial carcinoma treated with oral doses of MPA (Provera®) 150 mg/day the objective remission rate was 51%. The average duration of remissions obtained by MPA therapy was 14 months. The mean survival reaches 20 months in the subgroup of more hormone-responsive cases (15).

TABLE 5. *Endometrial adenocarcinoma[a]*

Residual cancer in operative specimen	MPA Silastic device application (%)	Radium packing (%)
No	59	62
With drug or radiation effect	8	14
Apparently viable	33	24

[a]Stage I without myometrial invasion: comparison between the efficiency of preoperative radiumpacking and preoperative intrauterine medroxyprogesterone silastic device application.

As the complete cure rate for *in situ* and stage I endometrial carcinoma using progestogens alone is only 60%, this hormone therapy is only indicated in selected cases, such as a carcinoma *in situ* in the endometrium of a younger woman still intending to have children. In stage I endometrial carcinoma, oral or parenteral progestogen therapy can be used as an adjuvant to radiosurgical treatment. Intrauterine insertion of a device impregnated with MPA replaces presurgical radiumpacking, therefore reducing the amount of exposure to radioactivity.

In advanced and recurrent endometrial carcinomas, administration of progestogens is the treatment of choice, can be complemented by radiotherapy, and never induces significant side effects.

Adjuvant Hormone Therapy

Progestogens are also used as adjuvants to the radiosurgical management of stage I endometrial carcinoma either prior to radium therapy or hysterectomy, or during the postoperative period (7).

Radical hysterectomy has, of course, a very important place in primary treatment of localized endometrial carcinoma. Preparing patients 4 weeks in advance of surgery by means of intrauterine radium-packing results in a 5-year survival rate of 72%. In a randomized study we have tried to evaluate the contribution of three different types of progestogen prophylaxis.

1. The first type of progestogen prophylaxis consisted of 1 g MPA/week during 4 weeks prior to radium-packing and increased the 5-year survival rate in this group to 90%. MPA makes the tumor more sensitive to ionizing radiation and therefore potentiates the effect of radiotherapy (19). Pathological examination of resected material reveals a significant decrease of apparently viable carcinomatous tissue in patients receiving progestogen adjuvant therapy as compared with those treated with radiation and surgery alone.

2. In the second type of progestogen prophylaxis we administered 1 g MPA/week during the 2 years following radium-packing and hysterectomy to prevent recurrences and metastatic dissemination. This approach resulted in an increase of the 5-year survival rate to 86%.

3. Finally, progestogen therapy prior to radium-packing followed by postsurgical progestogen prophylaxis yielded a 5-year survival rate of nearly 100%.

In a retrospective study we evaluated the influence of adjuvant progestogen therapy on the recurrence rate and the 5-year survival rate of patients treated with different therapeutic regimens. The recurrence rate, after correction for death from intercurrent disease, remained zero and the 5-year survival rate 100% (Fig. 5) (9).

Adjuvant progestogen treatment also seems to be effective in advanced (III–IV) stages (6). The objective remission rate achieved by radiotherapy alone (25%) and by MPA treatment alone (51%) was increased to 91% in a selected patient group by a combination of radiotherapy and MPA. In this way the average duration of remissions of the hormone-sensitive cases can be extended to 25 months, and the mean survival to 26 months.

The factors influencing the response of endometrial carcinoma to progestogen therapy can be divided into two groups: (a) those relating to the administration of the hormonal compound; and (b) those relating to the responsiveness of the tumor and the host. Moreover, these factors have a prognostic value, permitting monitoring of the response during the treatment.

Response to progestogens is conditioned by the type of drug, its route of administration, the dose, and the duration of treatment. These factors will determine progestogen levels in the serum.

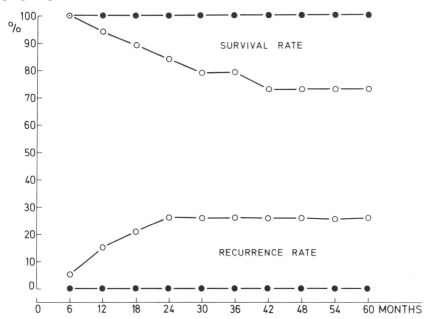

FIG. 5. Endometrial adenocarcinoma—Stage I. Seventy-one patients treated with radium therapy and/or hysterectomy. *Open circles:* without adjuvant therapy; *closed circles:* with adjuvant MPA therapy. Corrected for deaths from intercurrent disease.

Type of Drug

The mean objective remission rate obtained with progestogen compounds most frequently used to treat advanced or recurrent carcinoma proves their effectiveness against this type of cancer. Pure progesterone gives the best responses, but as a sufficient dose in oily solution cannot be injected, the practical superiority of MPA for cancer therapy remains evident (Table 6). Using the same dose of 1 g/week, oral administration achieved a 53% objective remission rate in the advanced disease compared with 31% by intramuscular injection. However, stage I endometrial carcinoma seems to respond better to intrauterine instillation of progestogen than to oral or parenteral administration.

Route of Administration

In our experience, the serum level of the administered progestogen correlates with the influence on the tumor cells. With MPA therapy, serum levels greater than 90 ng/ml radioimmunoassayable MPA are necessary to obtain a good response (8). With oral MPA treatment, serum MPA levels rise above 90 ng/ml within 10 days. With intramuscular administration it takes 5 weeks for MPA serum levels to reach the 90 ng/ml threshold (12,22). During intrauterine administration of MPA the serum MPA levels remain extremely low (< 10 ng/ml). This underlines the importance of the local cancerocidal mechanism of MPA.

Dose

Although many reports suggest that better results are obtained with a higher dose of progestogen and advocate very high "loading doses" during the first weeks of treatment, our survey on the effect of increasing doses of progesterone, MPA, and 17 α-OHPC on the remission rates did not indicate a direct dose-response relationship.

Duration of Treatment

Progestogen therapy should be continued for as long as the remission lasts; when MPA treatment is stopped striking relapses are often observed. Continuous admin-

TABLE 6. *Treatment of advanced or recurrent endometrial adenocarcinoma with progestogens*

Type of progestogen	Mean significant remission rate (%)	Number of reports
Progesterone	56	4
MPA	47	22
6,17α-dimethyl-6 dehydro-progesterone	33	4
17α-OHPC	28	15

istration of progestogen should also be made a rule for adjuvant therapy in order to avoid the risk of sudden recurrence.

Side Effects

Although progestogen therapy has been based on very high doses, which have, in some instances, been administered for long periods, we have never observed any significant hepatic, thrombotic, steroid, or mammary side effects. Both retrospective and prospective mammographic studies have provided evidence for the innocuous nature of MPA (10,13).

Good responsiveness of endometrial carcinoma to MPA is characterized by an objective tumor regression, as assessed clinically or radiologically, within 4–6 weeks of treatment, provided serum MPA levels reach at least 90 ng/ml. This responsiveness is directly related to the hormone dependency of the carcinoma and to the metabolic and hormonal status of the patient.

There is a general agreement on the prognostic value of some characteristics of the tumor (4,5,18). Well-differentiated carcinomas tend to show the best response. In patients with advanced or recurrent cancers it is the slowly growing primary or disseminated lesions which show the most dramatic remissions. In our experience, carcinomas with a primary endocervical origin are very sensitive to progestogens. The location of the tumor mass influences its responsiveness. Mobile vaginal recurrences and pulmonary and lymphatic metastases seem to be very responsive, while pelvic and abdominal tumors hardly respond at all. The type of primary treatment seems to have little influence on the results of subsequent progestogen therapy.

From our MPA study we were able to define the host factors favoring clinical response by the tumor (4,5,18). Older patients tend to be the best responders. Obesity, diabetes, and a high estrogen environment (all of which affect the hormonal and metabolic environment of the tumor) seem to indicate a good remission rate (Table 7).

TABLE 7. *Disseminated or recurrent uterine adenocarcinoma[a]*

Predictive factors		Significant remission rate (%)
Belonging to the tumor	⌠ Good differentiation	60
	⌡ Vaginal mobile tumor	65
Belonging to the host	⌠ Obesity	75
	⎬ Diabetes	71
	⌡ Vaginal smear K.I. ⩾ 5%	60
Mean reference rate		51

[a]115 cases treated by means of 1 gr medroxyprogesterone/week; preliminary predictive factors on hormone dependency and good responsiveness.

RESPONSE OF ENDOMETRIAL ADENOCARCINOMA TO ANTIESTROGENS

Antiestrogens block the estrogen receptor system and induce progestogen receptor synthesis, producing glycogen accumulation. The histological response is characterized by rapid transformation of pseudostratified carcinomatous glands to monolayered structures, consisting of high cylindrical and even atrophic cells with a low mitotic index which frequently exhibited atrophy and necrosis (1,28,34,41).

The addition of tamoxifen to the culture medium of organotypic cultures from endometrial adenocarcinomas induced the same histological transformations as observed *in vivo* in the treated patients. This was especially true for the transformation from pseudostratified to monolayered glandular structures. The essentially direct mechanism of action of tamoxifen on the endometrial adenocarcinoma cells affects their mitotic and secretory activity.

Under short- and long-term tamoxifen treatment serum estradiol levels remain at the menopausal level or fall to this level. This fall is characteristic in the responsive patient group. The serum estrone levels remain practically unchanged under tamoxifen treatment; nevertheless, in the responsive patient group, they tend to fall slightly (45). The serum FSH levels remain unchanged under tamoxifen treatment, while the LH levels remain unchanged or fall, if the initial values are within the higher menopausal range. All these hormonal data render an indirect mechanism of action for tamoxifen on endometrial adenocarcinoma quite improbable.

The vaginal smear of most adenocarcinoma patients under tamoxifen treatment remains or rapidly becomes estrogenic; this cytohormonal change is practically constant and seems to occur irrespective of any relationship to tumoral responsiveness for tamoxifen. In endometrial adenocarcinomas administration of tamoxifen induces a rapid and significant fall of estrogen receptor levels (Fig. 6) and an increase of cytosolic progestogen receptor levels (2,29,31,32,35–39) (Fig. 4).

From a therapeutic viewpoint, secondary tamoxifen treatment achieved over 50% objective regression rate in the 17 patients with persisting, recurrent, or metastatic endometrial adenocarcinoma, previously treated with MPA; 2 patients presented complete regression and 7 others partial regression with a mean duration of 3 months ranging between 2 and 5 months (Table 8). The clinical regression of the frequent vaginal recurrence of endometrial adenocarcinoma was rapidly induced; nevertheless malignant cells did not completely disappear in the vaginal smear of all responding patients. A close relationship was observed between the tumor responsiveness to MPA and to tamoxifen (26); the patients sensitive to tamoxifen were those who previously responded to MPA with a duration of remission of at least 3 months (Table 9). Under tamoxifen, the duration of the remission seemed markedly shorter.

As the majority of these persistent or recurrent endometrial adenocarcinomas were well or moderately differentiated and were localized to the vagina, no correlation could be made between differentiation or site of the tumor and its responsiveness to tamoxifen. Possible side effects (nausea, urticarial skin reaction) were observed in 2 patients, but disappeared after reducing the dose or stopping the treatment.

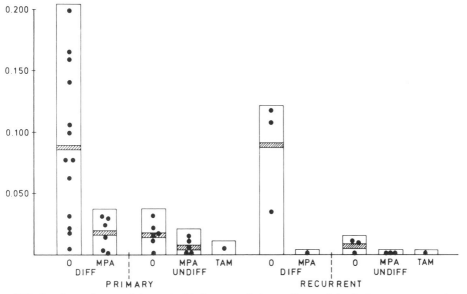

FIG. 6. Cytosolic estradiol receptor binding capacity in pmol/mg protein of primary or recurrent endometrial adenocarcinoma under MPA or tamoxifen treatment.

RESPONSE OF ENDOMETRIAL ADENOCARCINOMA TO ANTI-ESTROGEN–PROGESTOGEN COMBINATION

The rationale for this hormonal combination project in relation to endometrial adenocarcinoma is based on a possible manipulation of cytosolic estrogen and progestogen receptors in the tumor cells. From that viewpoint antiestrogens and progestogens both exert a double influence on the cytosolic steroid receptor system of the endometrial adenocarcinoma cells: a synergism by blocking the estrogen receptor system, and an antagonism towards the progestogen receptor, whose depletion is provoked by MPA and whose synthesis is induced by tamoxifen (16,40).

On an experimental basis we applied different types of tamoxifen–MPA combination therapy in the treatment of advanced, metastatic, or recurrent endometrial adenocarcinoma.

In a first trial, patients with a metastasis or a recurrence of a well or moderately differentiated, thus probably hormone-dependent, adenocarcinoma presenting paradoxically an atrophic or an intermediate vaginal smear, were treated by means of 40 mg tamoxifen per day by mouth until an estrogenic vaginal smear was induced. This priming of the adenocarcinoma cells was performed in order to enhance their responsiveness for MPA by inducing the synthesis of progesterone receptors and thus favoring the impact of the progestogens on the cell. This status is reached within a few weeks, so that the progestogen therapy (150 mg Provera® per day per os) can be successfully started.

In another trial, patients developing a metastasis or a recurrence during progestational adjuvant therapy for primary endometrial adenocarcinoma and those pre-

TABLE 8. *Response of advanced endometrial adenocarcinoma to successive MPA and tamoxifen treatment*

Patient	Histolog. Type	Response to MPA treatment		Response to tamoxifen treatment			
				Clinical		Cytological	
		Type	Duration	Type	Duration	PAP smear evolution	Cytohormonal evolution
75/1067	Diff.	Stabil.	4 m	Part. regres.	2 m	PAP V→PAP V	Atrophic→Estrog.
75/1117	Undiff.	Progres.	2 m	Stabil.	2 m	PAP V→PAP V	Subatr.→Estrog.
73/1136	Well diff.	Compl. regres.	6 m	Part. regres.	5 m	PAP V→PAP V	Atrophic→Subatr.
76/1247	Mod. diff.	Unsucc. adjuv.	6 m	Progres.	2 m	PAP II→PAP II	Subatr.→Estrog.
76/1048	Well diff.	Stabil.	4 m	Progres.	1½m	PAP V→PAP V	Atrophic→Atrophic
75/1706	Well diff.	Progres.	5 m	Stabil.	1 m	PAP V→PAP V	Subatr.→Estrog.
69/1151	Well diff.	Compl. regres.	9 y	{ Part. regres. / Stabil.	3 m / 5 m	PAP V→PAP I	
72/1618	Diff.	Compl. regres.	5 y	Part. regres.	1 m	PAP V→PAP V	Subatr.→Subatr.
77/1312	Mod. diff.	Unsucc. adjuv.	1 y	Stabil.	3 m	PAP V→PAP V	Subatr.→Estrog.
77/1156	Well diff.	I Adjuv.	1 y	{ Compl. regres. / Stabil.	2 m / 2 m	PAP V→PAP V	Atrophic→Estrog.
		II { Compl. regres. / Stabil.	3 m / 12 m	Compl. regres.	3 m		Atrophic→Estrog.
78/1140	Mixed + Clear cell	Unsucc. adjuv.	3 m / 3 m	Progres.	3 m.	PAP V→PAP III	Subatr.→Subatr.
78/1689	Mod. diff.	Stabil.	3 m	Part. regres.	2 m	PAP II→PAP I	Subatr.→Subatr.
73/0098	Diff.	Stabil.	5 y	Part. regres.	2 m	PAP III→PAP II	Atrophic→Atrophic
78/2004	Adenosq.	Unsucc. adjuv.	1 m	Progres.	1½m	PAP IV→PAP I	Subatr.→Estrog.
77/1617	Mod. diff. + Adeno acant.	Unsucc. adjuv.	1 m	Part. regres.	3 m	PAP V→PAP I	Estrog.→Subatr.
77/1793	Well diff.	Adjuv.	2 y	Compl. regres.	4 m	PAP I→PAP I	Subatr.→Estrog.
77/1079	Undiff.	Adjuv.	1½y	Stabil.	2 m	PAP I→PAP I	Estrog.→Estrog.

TABLE 9. *Relationship between the responses of advanced endometrial adenocarcinoma to successive MPA and tamoxifen treatment*

Response to 1° line MPA treatment		Response to 2° line tamoxifen treatment			
		Complete regression	Partial regression	Stabilization	Progression
Complete regression	4	1	3		
Stabilization	4		3		1
Adjuvant therapy	2	1		1	
Unsuccessful adjuvant therapy	4		1		3
Total	14	2	7	1	4

senting a relapse after a significant regression of a first metastasis or recurrence under MPA therapy, are previously submitted to a 2-week 40-mg/day tamoxifen regimen before starting again the progestational therapy for another 2 weeks. At that moment, a second line sequential antiestrogen–progestogen treatment is realized.

In a last trial, the same patient groups are treated with a combined 40 mg tamoxifen—150 mg Provera a day regimen. Thus, tamoxifen corroborates the blocking of the estrogen receptor system by medroxyprogesterone and moreover, guarantees the replenishment of the adenocarcinoma cells with progestogen receptors, consumed by the incorporated medroxyprogesterone.

REFERENCES

1. Armstrong, E. M., and More, I. A. R. (1974): *Cytobios*, 11:13–16.
2. Bichon, M., and Bayard, F. (1979): *Ann. Endocrinol.*, 40:43–44.
3. Billiet, G., Bonte, J., and Ide, P. (1971): In: *Basic Actions of Sex Steroids on Target Organs*, edited by P. O. Hubinont, F. Leroy, and P. Galand, pp. 280–283. Kargel, Basel.
4. Bonte, J. (1972): *Cancro*, XXV:11–15.
5. Bonte, J. (1972): *Acta Obstet. Gynecol. Scand (Suppl.)*, 19:21–24.
6. Bonte, J. (1973): In: *Symposium on Endometrial Cancer*, edited by M. G. Brush, R. W. Taylor, and D. C. Williams, pp. 203–211. Heinemann, London.
7. Bonte, J. (1974): *Méd. Hyg.*, 1107:1106–1107.
8. Bonte, J. (1975): *Méd. Hyg.*, 1173:1831.
9. Bonte, J. (1977): *Méd. Hyg.*, 35:4193–4197.
10. Bonte, J. (1977): In: *Gynecology and Obstetrics, (Excerpta Medica Int. Congr. Series, no. 412)*, pp. 139–154. Excerpta Medica, Amsterdam.
11. Bonte, J. (1978): In: *Hormonal Biology of Endometrial Cancer, (U.I.C.C. Technical Report Series, Vol. 42)*, edited by G. S. Richardson and D. T. MacLaughlin, pp. 155–187. I.U.C.C., Geneva.
12. Bonte, J. (1978): *Gynaek. Rundsch.*, 18:172–182.
13. Bonte, J. (1978): *Gynaek. Rundsch.*, 18:220–245.
14. Bonte, J. (1979): *Rev. Endocrinol. Related Cancer*, 3:11–17.
15. Bonte, J. (1980): In: *Hormones and Cancer*, edited by S. Jacobelli, R. J. B. King, H. R. Lindner, and M. E. Lippman, pp. 443–455. Raven Press, New York.
16. Bonte, J. (1980): In: *Progestogens in the Management of Hormone Responsive Cancers*, edited by R. W. Taylor, pp. 35–49, The Medicine Publishing Foundation, Oxford.
17. Bonte, J., De Coster, J. M., and Billiet, G. (1978): *Gynecol. Oncol.*, 6:60–75.

18. Bonte, J., De Coster, J. M., Drochmans, A., Ide, P., and Billiet, G. (1970): *C. R. Soc. Franç. Gynécol.*, 1:1–7.
19. Bonte, J., De Coster, J. M., and Ide, P. (1970): *Cancer*, 25(4):907–910.
20. Bonte, J., De Coster, J. M., and Ide, P. (1977): *Acta Cytol.*, 21:218–224.
21. Bonte, J., De Coster, J. M., Ide, P., and Billiet, G. (1978): In: *Endometrial Cancer*, edited by M. G. Brush, R. B. J. King, and R. W. Taylor, pp. 192–205. Baillière-Tindall, London.
22. Bonte, J., De Coster, J. M., Ide, P., Wynants, P., and Billiet, G. (1974): In: *Recent Progress in Obstetrics and Gynaecology (Excerpta Medica Int. Congr. Series, no. 329)*, edited by L. S. Persianinov, T. V. Chervakova, and J. Presl, pp. 285–297. Excerpta Medica, Amsterdam.
23. Bonte, J., Drochmans, A., and Ide, P. (1966): *Acta Obstet. Gynecol. Scand.*, 45:121–129.
24. Bonte, J., Drochmans, A., and Ide, P. (1966): *Excerpta Medica Found. Int. Congr. Ser.*, no. 111:307.
25. Bonte, J., Drochmans, A., and Lassance, M. (1966): *Gynécol. Obstet. (Paris)*, 65(2):179–185.
26. Bonte, J., Ide, P., Billiet, G., and Wynants, P. (1981): *Gynecol. Oncol.*, 11:140–161.
27. De Coster, J. M., Bonte, J., and Marcq, A. (1977): *Gynecol. Oncol.*, 5:189–195.
28. El-Sheikha, Z., Klopper, A., and Beck, J. S. (1972): *Clin. Endocrinol.*, 1:275–282.
29. Fromson, J. M., and Sharp, D. S. (1974): *J. Obstet. Gynaecol. Br. Commonw.*, 81:321–323.
30. Ide, P., and Bonte, J. (1974): *Br. J. Cancer*, 30:175 (abstr.)
31. Jordan, V. C., and Dowse, L. J. (1976): *J. Endocrinol.*, 68:297–303.
32. Jordan, V. C., and Koerner, S. (1975): *Eur. J. Cancer*, 11:205–207.
33. Kelley, R. M., and Baker, W. H. (1961): *N. Engl. J. Med.*, 264:216–222.
34. Kistner, R. W. (1965): *Obstet. Gynecol. Surv.*, 20:873–897.
35. Koseki, Y., Zava, D. T., Chamness, G. C., and McGuire, W. L. (1977): *Steroids*, 30:169–177.
36. Legha, S., and Muggia, F. M. (1976): *Ann. Intern. Med.*, 84:751.
37. Lunan, C. B., and Green, G. (1973): *Biochem. Soc. Trans.*, 1:500–502.
38. Lunan, C. B., and Green, B. (1974): *Clin. Endocrinol.*, 3:465–480.
39. Robel, P., Levy, C., Wolfe, J. P., Nicolas, J. C., and Baulieu, E. E. (1978): *C. R. Acad. Sci.*, 278:1353–1357.
40. Sekiya, G., and Takamizawa, H. (1975): *Br. J. Obstet. Gynaecol.*, 82:80–83.
41. Sherman, B. M., Chapler, F. K., Crickard, K. A., and Wycoff, D. (1978): *Clin. Res.*, 26(5):703.
42. Swenerton, K. D., Shaw, D., White, G. D., and Boyes, D. A. (1979):*N. Engl. J. Med.*, 30(2):105.
43. Tisman, G., Kellon, D. B., Wu, S., and Safiro, G. E. (1976): *Clin. Res.*, 24(3):381 *(abstr.)*.
44. Wall, J. A., Franklin, R. R., Kaufman, R. H., et al. (1965): *Am. J. Obstet. Gynecol.*, 99:842–849.
45. Watson, J., Alain, M., Anderson, F. B., and Heald, P. J. (1974): *Biochem. Soc. Trans.*, 2:982–983.
46. Wolff, E., and Wolff, E. (1966): *Eur. J. Cancer*, 2:93–103.

Role of Medroxyprogesterone in Endocrine-
Related Tumors, Volume II, edited by L.
Campio, G. Robustelli Della Cuna, and R. W.
Taylor. Raven Press, New York © 1983.

The Treatment of Endometrial Carcinoma with Medroxyprogesterone Acetate

R. W. Taylor

*Department of Obstetrics and Gynaecology, St. Thomas's Hospital Medical School,
London SE1 7EH, United Kingdom*

Most clinicians take an optimistic view of the results they obtain by treating endometrial carcinoma by surgery with adjuvant radiotherapy. There are many reports of cure rates above 80% when the growth is confined to the uterus at the time of operation (8,17). However, the overall cure rate is no more than 55–60% (6), which closely resembles that for carcinoma of the cervix, generally believed to be a much more virulent tumor. Clearly, the results for advanced tumors, treated by conventional methods are less than satisfactory. Furthermore, most advanced lesions are not suitable for a surgical approach and radiotherapy is the method of choice. If this fails, there is little scope for further treatment because normal tissues adjacent to the malignancy have already received the maximum dose of radiation. Not surprisingly therefore, there has been an extensive search for alternative methods of treatment. Conventional chemotherapy, using powerful antimetabolites or metabolic antagonists are not very successful and their side effects generally outweigh the benefits they confer. Hormone therapy, on the other hand, offers in theory at least considerable advantages.

Endometrial carcinoma arises in what is probably the prime estrogen target tissue. Sensitivity to estrogen can be measured by counting molecules of receptor protein in the cytoplasm (12,19) and it is found that all endometrial carcinomas contain this receptor to some degree (19). The quantity of receptor protein does vary with the degree of differentiation of the tumor (20), but as the majority of patients with endometrial carcinoma have relatively well-differentiated tumors, we are most often dealing with a malignancy that responds to both estrogen stimulation and estrogen deprivation.

Progesterone, the natural hormone secreted during the luteal phase of the menstrual cycle, is in many ways an estrogen antagonist—both generally and specifically within the estrogen target tissues. It does, for example, counter the salt- and water-retaining properties of estrogen and it converts a watery, profuse cervical mucus to a scanty, viscous fluid. More important in the present context it largely puts a stop to proliferation in the endometrium. It induces a change in the secretory pattern of the epithelial cells and an increase in rate of division of stromal cells. The action of progesterone in the endometrium depends upon prior stimulation by estrogen because the development of progesterone receptors is controlled by estrogen (3). In theory, therefore, endometrial carcinoma should be inhibited by progesterone and the better differentiated tumors should respond better than those that are poorly differentiated.

There are two broad approaches to the use of hormones in managing endometrial carcinoma. They may be used in the treatment of late disease, largely in palliation, or they may be used as adjuvants to conventional surgery and radiotherapy, early in treatment in an attempt to prevent small metastases and even isolated malignant cells split at operation from developing into large tumors. There are many reports of the value of hormones in the treatment of late disease, but I have been forced to rely largely upon the experience of the unit at St. Thomas' Hospital when trying to judge the value of adjuvant therapy.

Based upon an understanding of the physiological response of normal endometrium to the sex steroids, it is clear that the first line of approach to the treatment of endometrial malignancy is the removal of the uterus and of estrogen stimulation. This latter is usually accomplished in large part by removing the ovaries surgically or destroying them by radiotherapy. However, there is inevitably some estrogen produced by the adrenal glands, or by peripheral conversion of adrenal androgens by fatty tissues, and so some form of progesterone/progestogen therapy is needed in addition. In theory, the progesterone sensitivity of an endometrial carcinoma could be enhanced by prior treatment with estrogen. This would seem to be particularly applicable to patients who are long postmenopausal, but so far there are no good reports in which this approach has been tried. In view of the known liking of such tumors for estrogen it is easy to understand the reluctance of clinicians to take the risks involved. Estrogen antagonists such as clomiphene and tamoxiphen could have the advantage of increasing progesterone sensitivity without necessarily stimulating growth. A limited amount of personal experience to date suggests that this approach deserves more attention than it has had so far.

PROGESTOGENS IN ADVANCED DISEASE

Kelly and Baker (9,10) produced the first report of progestogen therapy in extensive disease, showing that regression can be caused in localized and metastatic carcinoma. Briggs et al. (2) reviewed 822 cases from the literature reporting that 31.3% (256 cases) showed objective remission. Many other studies since have shown a similar remission rate. All agree that the better differentiated primary tumors show the best remission rate. Occasionally the remission appears to be complete and lasts for many years. In treating 20 patients with extensive recurrent disease at St. Thomas's Hospital we had measurable remission in 6 patients. Two of these patients were well and apparently tumor-free 5 years after beginning treated with 100 mg medroxyprogesterone acetate three times daily. In the other cases where there was remission, the relief lasted for between 3 and 24 months. After a time there was further development of the tumor and eventually all of these patients died of their disease. In no case was any ill effect of the progestogen seen. Some patients derived a sense of well-being which was possibly related to the mild cortico-steroid effect of the hormone (14).

PROGESTOGENS AS ADJUNCTS TO OTHER TREATMENTS IN EARLY DISEASE

Surgery used alone in the treatment of endometrial carcinoma that appears to be confined to the body of the uterus gives good results when compared with other forms of malignancy, but not good enough. Rickford (18) showed that in such cases there was a 5.5% unexpected involvement of pelvic lymph nodes, but this still leaves 15% of patients who clearly have microscopic spread of the disease at the time of operation, for the best reported results show a 20% recurrence rate within 5–10 years. As most recurrent growth is initially confined to the pelvis (13) local radiotherapy either before or after surgery should be helpful. Certainly this appears to be the case in stage II disease (FIGO classification), but when there is evidence of only superficial invasion of the myometrium the addition of radiotherapy to surgery does not seem to improve the 5-year survival (5,7,8,15,16).

Clearly there is a potential value in an adjuvant, and theoretically a progestational agent, administered systemically, could be the drug we are seeking. Many workers have shown the value of locally applied progestogens (4,11), but as it is the spread of cells beyond the uterus that concerns us, systemic administration seems to be most appropriate. As the drug has to be given for some months, or even years in some cases, oral administration is preferable to injection. With oral administration of medroxyprogesterone acetate, it is possible to produce serum levels above 90 ng/ml within 10 days, whereas it takes 5 weeks to achieve the same levels with intramuscular administration. The level we should aim to achieve in dealing with endometrial carcinoma appears to be 90 ng/ml (1).

With these considerations in mind, the manner of treating carcinoma of the body of the uterus was changed at St. Thomas' Hospital 11 years ago. The prime treatment remained hysterectomy and bilateral salpingo-oophorectomy with or without pre- or postoperative radiotherapy according to the decision of individual clinicians in individual cases. The sole change in policy was the addition of medroxyprogesterone acetate orally in a dose of 300 mg per day from the time of the first diagnostic curettage when there was a reasonable suspicion that the patient had an endometrial carcinoma. If the diagnosis was not confirmed by histological examination the drug was stopped. If the diagnosis was confirmed, the major treatment was decided upon and carried out. The drug was maintained for 6 weeks in the absence of evidence of pelvic spread at laparotomy. If there was evidence of such spread, it was main-tained indefinitely.

THE ST. THOMAS EXPERIENCE (1970–1980)

There were a total of 130 patients. The age range was from 39 to 82, with a mean age of 56. One-quarter of all the patients were premenopausal. The stage of the tumor at presentation is shown in Table 1. During the 30 years we have been keeping careful records there has been a steady increase in the proportion of patients with early disease.

Using information from the study of Metters and Milton it is possible to calculate an "expected" death rate for the 10-year period. For example, because there were 10 patients with stage I disease in 1970 and the death rate for stage I disease in the Unit was 10% over 10 years, we would have expected 1 death among the 1970 group of patients. I realize the difficulties involved in this sort of calculation, but as patients have been added to the study throughout the decade and indeed are still being added, it will be another 10 years before absolute 10-year survival times for the whole group are known. Table 2 shows the histological grading of the tumors.

The survival rate and recurrence rate in the 130 patients treated with adjuvant medroxyprogesterone acetate, against expected rates, are shown in Fig. 1. There were 28 deaths from intercurrent disease in patients who as far as was known did not have recurrent carcinoma. Unfortunately only four post-mortem examinations were available so it can not be certain that there were no recurrences among the group.

So far there have been no deaths from recurrent endometrial carcinoma when medroxyprogesterone acetate was added to what was thought to be curative surgery or radiotherapy. On the basis of past experience we would have expected 8 deaths during the decade in this group of patients.

There has been 1 patient only who is known to have developed a recurrence. She had poorly differentiated growth, which was in the fundus of the uterus, invading the myometrium only to a depth of 1–2 mm and in the normal course of events would have received treatment by surgery alone plus medroxyprogesterone acetate. At a routine examination 3 months after operation she was found to have some small vault granulations which, on histological examination, proved to be poorly differentiated adenocarcinoma. She was given radiotherapy by local application to the vaginal vault and has remained free of further recurrence during the past 4 years.

TABLE 1. *Distribution of cases by stage of tumor with calculated "expected deaths"*

	Nos.	%	Expected deaths
Stage I	97	74.6	4
Stage II	29	22.3	2
Stage III	2	1.5	1
Stage IV	2	1.5	1

TABLE 2. *Histological differential of tumors*

Poorly differentiated	12%
Moderately well differentiated	24%
Well differentiated	64%

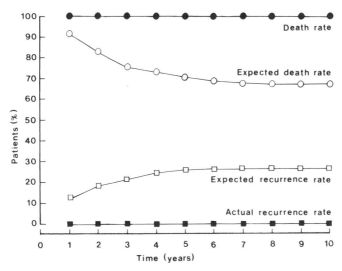

FIG. 1. The survival rate and recurrence rate in 130 patients treated with adjuvant medroxyprogesterone acetate against expected rates.

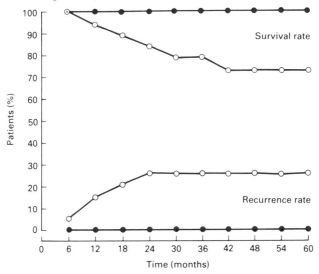

FIG. 2. Survival rate and recurrence rate of 71 patients with stage I endometrial carcinoma treated with radium-therapy and/or hysterectomy with *(closed circles)* or without *(open circles)* adjuvant medroxyprogesterone acetate. Corrected for deaths from intercurrent disease. (From Bonte, ref. 1, with permission.)

Bonte (1) published a report of survival and recurrence rates in patients treated by conventional surgery and radiotherapy with and without adjuvant medroxyprogesterone acetate (Fig. 2). This, like our study, shows extremely encouraging results. New studies on the induction of specific enzymes which are concerned with the mechanism of steroid hormone action in the endometrium offer the hope of being able to mount shorter term studies than have previously been practicable (12). Our experiments show that these enzymes are induced in endometrial carcinoma within 24 hr of starting treatment with oral medroxyprogesterone acetate. Meanwhile it seems to me that the use of surgery/radiotherapy and adjuvant medroxyprogesterone acetate should be regarded as offering the best available treatment in the light of current knowledge.

REFERENCES

1. Bonte, J. (1980): In: *Progesterone in the Management of Hormone Responsive Carcinomas*, edited by R. W. Taylor, p. 35. The Medicine Publishing Foundation, Oxford, United Kingdom.
2. Briggs, M. H., Caldwell, A. D. S., and Pitchford, A. G. (1967): *Hospital Med.*, 2:63.
3. Crocker, S. G., Milton, P. J. D., Taylor, R. W., and King, R. J. B. (1975): In: *Gynaecological Malignancy*, edited by M. G. Brush and R. W. Taylor, p. 179. Bailliere Tindall, London.
4. Decoster, J. M., Bonte, J., and Marcq, A. (1977): *Gynecol. Oncol.*, 5:189.
5. Frick, H. C., Munnell, E. W., Richart, R. M., Berger, A. P., and Lawry, M. F. (1973): *Am. J. Obstet. Gynecol.*, 115:663.
6. Gusberg, S. B., and Yannopoulos, D. (1964): *Am. J. Obstet. Gynecol.*, 88:157.
7. Joelsson, I., Levine, R. U., and Moberger, G. (1971): *Am. J. Obstet. Gynecol.*, 111:696.
8. Jones, W. E., Kanner, H. M., Kanner, H. H., and Benson, C. (1972): *Am. J. Obstet. Gynecol.*, 113:549.
9. Kelly, R. M., and Baker, W. M. (1959): *Conference on Experimental Cancer Chemotherapy*, Monograph 9,p.235. National Cancer Institute, Bethesda, Maryland.
10. Kelly, R. M., and Baker, W. M. (1970): In: *Progress in Gynaecology*, edited by S. M. Sturgis and M. L. Taymor, p. 362. Grune & Stratton, New York.
11. Kettle, M. J., and Melch, D. H. (1972): In: *Symposium on Endometrial Cancer*, edited by M. G. Brush, R. W. Taylor, and D. C. Williams, p. 237. Heinemann, London.
12. King, R. J. B., Brush, M. G., and Taylor, R. W. (1973): In: *Symposium on Endometrial Cancer*, edited by M. G. Brush, R. W. Taylor, and D. C. Williams, p. 165. Heinemann, London.
13. Long, R. T., Sala, J. M., and Spratt, J. S. (1972): *Cancer*, 29:318.
14. MacDonald, R. R. (1972): In: *Symposium on Endometrial Cancer*, edited by M. G. Brush, R. W. Taylor, and D. C. Williams, p. 212. Heinemann, London.
15. McGarrity, K. A., and Scott, G. C. (1968): *J. Obstet. Gynaecol. Br. Commonw.*, 75:455.
16. Milton, P. J. D., and Metters, J. S. (1972): *J. Obstet. Gynaecol. Br. Commonw.*, 79:455.
17. Nilsen, P. A., and Kolstad, P. (1973): In: *Symposium on Endometrial Cancer*, edited by M. G. Brush, R. W. Taylor, and D. C. Williams, p. 115. Heinemann, London.
18. Rickford, R. B. K. (1968): *J. Obstet. Gynaecol. Br. Commonw.*, 75:580.
19. Taylor, R. W. (1964): *J. Obstet. Gynaecol. Br. Commonw.*, 81:163.
20. Taylor, R. W. (1979): *Am. J. Obstet. Gynecol.*, 132:61.

Role of Medroxyprogesterone in Endocrine-Related Tumors, Volume II, edited by L. Campio, G. Robustelli Della Cuna, and R. W. Taylor. Raven Press, New York © 1983.

A Controlled Clinical Trial on Stage I Endometrial Carcinoma: Rationale and Methodological Approach

G. De Palo, *C. Mangioni, **P. Periti,
M. Merson, and M. Del Vecchio

*National Cancer Institute of Milan, Milan; *I Department of Obstetrics and Gynecology, University of Milan, Milan; and **Department of Pharmacology, University of Florence, Florence, Italy*

The survival rates (absolute survival and relapse-free survival) of patients with FIGO stage I endometrial carcinoma, the most frequent stage of this disease, have a wide range. These are dependent on prognostic factors, clinical or pathologic stage, type of treatment, and general conditions of the patients.

Many factors have been identified that appear to have predictive value in patients with endometrial carcinoma. Some of them are definite, others probable. The first group includes histologic differentiation, myometrial invasion, retroperitoneal (pelvic and para-aortic) node metastases. The second group includes positive peritoneal cytology, histologic type (adenocarcinoma, adenoacanthoma, clear cell carcinoma, adenosquamous carcinoma, undifferentiated carcinoma), and invasion of the intramural tract of the fallopian tube. The predictive value of the only prognostic factor taken into consideration by FIGO, the length of the uterine cavity, is negligible (1,2,11,27).

HISTOPATHOLOGIC GRADING

The degree of histologic differentiation is one of the most sensitive prognostic factors (1,2,27,28,42). The survival rate decreases with increasing histopathologic grading. In other words, G3 patients have a worse prognosis than G1 and G2 patients, whereas the difference between G1 and G2 is less important (11).

Histopathological grade is correlated with the depth of myometrial invasion (7). As the tumor becomes less differentiated, myometrial invasion increases (7,33).

MYOMETRIAL INVASION

The depth of myometrial invasion (M1, M2, M3) and the proximity of the invading tumor to the uterine serosa is another prognostic factor. A review of the literature clearly shows a decrease in 5-year survival as myometrial invasion increases (20). Lutz et al. (26) have demonstrated that patients whose tumors are more than 10 mm from the uterine serosa had a 5-year survival rate equal to 97%, whereas those with a tumor within 5 mm of the uterine serosa had a 65% survival rate.

RADIOLOGIC LYMPH NODE METASTASES

Contrary to cervical and ovarian carcinomas, very little interest has been shown for the routine clinical use of lymphography in endometrial carcinoma.

In the retrospective study of the Istituto Nazionale Tumori of Milan and the First Department of Obstetrics and Gynecology of the University of Milan, 182 new cases with histologically proven endometrial carcinoma were evaluated with lymphography. The incidence of abnormal lymphograms according to clinical and pathologic stage (all the available diagnostic criteria except the evaluation of the retroperitoneal node chains) was 8.9% in clinical and 8% pathologic stage I (Table 1). The results of our series correlate with the results of Kademian et al. (21), and both are remarkably inferior to those of others. This is due to the fact that in our report, as well as in that of Kademian et al., pathologic stage grouping has been used for a large case material. In other reports, where a clinical classification has been used, an initial understaging of the patients can explain the higher incidence of metastases in the early stages (10,12,15,16,32,44).

The overall diagnostic accuracy (radiologic-histologic correlation) in both the 51 positive and negative, previously untreated patients was 86.3% (44/51 patients). The "specificity" (normal lymphographic percentage of histologically negative cases) was 91.4% (32/35) and the "sensitivity" (pathologic lymphographic percentage of histologically positive cases) 75% (12/16). There were three false-positive and four false-negative reports, and two of these patients had embolic micrometastases.

Lymphographic diagnostic accuracy is not completely satisfactory. There could be two reasons for this: first, the lymph nodes of aged women present extensive · fatty and fibrous changes, which make the diagnosis difficult; second, the lack of experience of radiologists with this disease.

As regards the site of metastases according to the literature (18,38,39,44) there are three draining trunks from the body of the uterus. The first drains along the

TABLE 1. *Incidence of retroperitoneal metastases as disclosed by lymphography in stage I endometrial carcinoma*

Staging modality	Author	% of nodal metastases
Clinical	Gerteis	20.0
	Musumeci et al.	10.9
Pathological	Kademian et al.	12.8
	Musumeci et al.	8.0

gonadal vessels to the para-aortic nodes, the second runs via the parametria to the external and common iliac nodes, and the third follows the round ligament and goes to the superficial inguinal nodes. Anatomically, the first one seems to be the major pathway of the uterine corpus.

In our series (31), the pelvic nodes, alone (56.2%) or in combination with the para-aortic (34.3%), were the more frequently compromised.

On the basis of these results, the "anatomic" predominance of the ovarian pedicle is not confirmed, but on the contrary, lymphatic drainage through the anatomically secondary parametrial channels seems to be the most important for dissemination of the disease.

HISTOLOGIC LYMPH NODE METASTASES

The remote literature has shown an incidence of lymph node metastases ranging from 5% (22,40) to 23% (41) in patients at FIGO stage I submitted to pelvic lymph node biopsies. In a review of the literature performed by Morrow et al. (29), of 369 patients with FIGO stage I endometrial carcinoma 39 had metastases to the pelvic lymph nodes. In the more recent series of Creasman et al. (8), of 140 patients 16 had positive pelvic nodes (11.6%). Summing up the results of remote and recent literature, 60/602 patients with FIGO stage I endometrial carcinoma had pelvic node metastases (9.9%) (Table 2).

The incidence of metastases correlates well with the histopathologic grade of the tumor, and the depth of myometrial invasion.

As regards the incidence of para-aortic metastases, controversial data have been reported. Creasman et al. (8) found that in 102 of 140 patients in whom the para-aortic chains were histologically examined, 10 (9.8%) had metastases. In the analysis of further data of the Gynecologic Oncology Group (GOG) protocol, 23 of 206 patients with FIGO stage I endometrial carcinoma had pelvic node metastases; 75% of 23 patients had para-aortic node sampling, and 16 of these had metastases

TABLE 2. *Incidence of pelvic node metastases in*
FIGO stage I endometrial carcinoma

Authors	Patient ratio (%)
Liu and Meigs (1955)	4/33 (12.0)
Schwartz and Brunschwig (1957)	2/14 (14.0)
Roberts (1961)	5/22 (23.0)
Hawksworth (1964)	8/64 (12.5)
Rickford (1968)	2/36 (5.0)
Lees (1969)	3/56 (5.0)
Lewis (1970)	12/107 (11.0)
Homesley (1976/77)	8/130 (6.0)
Creasman (1976)	16/140 (9.9)
Total	60/602 (9.9)

in the para-aortic nodes (9,13). Nevertheless, it is not clear if the reported metastases were para-aortic alone or para-aortic plus pelvic.

It seems that in the data of the literature, the true incidence of lymph node metastases is limited to the pelvic chains, contemporaneously involving the pelvic and aortic nodes or limited to the para-aortic region, is confusing.

The presence of nodal metastases is the major prognostic factor. The following data are significant. Morrow et al. (29) in their review of the literature reported that only 31% of those patients with stage I disease and positive pelvic nodes survived 5 years, and most of these had been treated with postoperative radiotherapy. In the study of the National Cancer Institute and "Mangiagalli" I Department of Obstetrics and Gynecology (31), the group of patients with pathologic stage I and II disease without lymphographically proven metastases had a 5-year survival rate of 78% compared with 54% for patients with retroperitoneal involvement ($p = 0.05$). It is noteworthy that the patients with positive lymph nodes received external radiotherapy (45-50 Gy) on the pelvis with or without para-aortic areas.

SURGICAL STAGING AND SURGICAL TREATMENT

Intensive surgical staging of the disease changes the stage in a large percentage of patients. In fact, understaging FIGO classification versus pathologic classification is about 15–20%.

Total abdominal hysterectomy with bilateral salpingo-oophorectomy plus colpectomy of the superior third of the vagina and selective retroperitoneal node biopsies is the surgical treatment of choice.

RADIOTHERAPY

With adequate attention to irradiation of the vaginal vault, and with intracavitary radium techniques or external high voltage therapy, the incidence of vaginal persistence after surgery can be diminished significantly as compared with that obtained with surgery alone (6). Pelvic recurrence (central and/or nodal) is significantly diminished by the use of external high voltage radiotherapy on the pelvis after surgery.

ADJUVANT HORMONE THERAPY

It is well known that the progestogens, more than chemotherapeutic agents, are useful in the treatment of advanced or recurrent endometrial carcinoma (36). Their utility in increasing radiosensitivity and in diminishing the recurrence rate, when administered before radiotherapy or surgery, has been also established (3–5).

The effectiveness of progestogens as adjuvant hormone therapy is still unknown. A randomized clinical trial on 574 cases treated with adjuvant progestogens versus placebo treatment showed no significant contribution to survival by adjuvant hormone therapy (24). On the contrary, a pilot study performed at the National Cancer Institute of Milan (11) suggested a possible influence of prolonged adjuvant hormone treatment on the extension of survival and the percentage of survivors free of tumor in FIGO stage I endometrial carcinoma with depth myometrial invasion.

For all the above-mentioned reasons the subproject "Clinical Multimodality Therapy," of the Applications-Oriented Project "Control of Neoplastic Growth" of the National Research Council of Italy, undertook in 1980 a controlled study on this disease.

THE AIM AND DESIGN OF THE CONTROLLED STUDY

The aim of the study was threefold: (a) to perform in patients with FIGO stage I endometrial carcinoma a complete presurgical and surgical staging and to establish the conversion rate from clinical to pathologic stage; (b) to establish a treatment plan (surgery alone, surgery plus external high voltage therapy) on the basis of pathologic extension of the disease; (c) to establish the effectiveness of adjuvant hormone therapy.

In addition to the clinical aim, other objectives are the study of estrogen-progesterone receptors in correlation with the natural history of the disease and the study of the pharmacokinetics of medroxyprogesterone acetate (MPA, Farmitalia). The design of the controlled study is illustrated in Fig. 1. All patients with FIGO stage I endometrial carcinoma (after fractional curettage) are registered.

Presurgical staging consists of chest X-ray, intravenous urography, foot lymphography, X-ray of pelvic bones, rectosigmoidoscopy and/or double contrast enema; liver scan is optional.

Surgical staging consists of peritoneal cytology (free fluid and peritoneal washing) performed as the first step during laparotomy; inspection of omentum and abdominal viscera with biopsies on suspected lesions; selective lymphadenectomy on pelvic and para-aortic nodes in the presence of pathologic lymphography or enlarged surgical lymph nodes.

The surgical treatment consists of total abdominal hysterectomy with bilateral salpingo-oophorectomy plus colpectomy of the superior third of the vagina.

On the basis of histopathologic grading, myometrial invasion and histologically positive pelvic or para-aortic nodes, the patients were stratified in three risk group levels. Other prognostic factors, i.e., histologic type, peritoneal cytology and "risk factors" according to Nolan (34,35), will be evaluated in the future.

The histopathologic grading system was achieved by using the classification which subdivides carcinoma into three groups: grade I, high degree of differentiation; grade II, medium degree of differentiation; grade III, low degree of differentiation or undifferentiated carcinoma. The maximum depth of tumor infiltration in the myometrium was the criterion used to divide the cases into four groups: M0, neoplasm confined to the endometrium without myometrial invasion; M1, tumor involving as much as one-third of the myometrium; M2, tumor involving as much as two-thirds of the myometrium; M3, tumor involving the whole thickness of the myometrium and reaching the serosa.

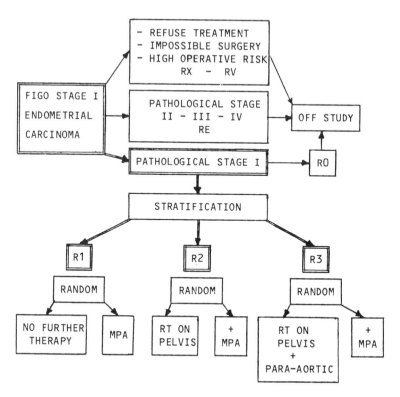

FIG. 1. Controlled clinical trial on stage I endometrial carcinoma—CNR 07179/N: Design of study.

All the definitive histologic specimens and peritoneal cytologic slides should be reviewed by the consultant pathologists, as all lymphangiograms should be reviewed by the consultant radiologists.

The risk group levels considered for the study are the following: R1, the G1-G2-M1 categories; R2, the G1-G2-M2-M3 or G3-M1-M2-M3 categories; R3, any G, any M, N+ categories.

The following groups of patients are not admitted to the study: age more than 75 years (in the course of the study the admission of patients was limited to age ≤75 years); geographic inaccessibility; previous treatment; previous or synchronous neoplastic disease with the exception of cutaneous epithelioma; patients who refuse a diagnostic work-up or postsurgical treatment; patients with mixed mesodermal tumor; patients with severe disease such as cardiovascular disturbances or neuro-psychiatric difficulties; patients not submitted to surgery for high operative risk or for refusal of surgical treatment; patients submitted to vaginal hysterectomy for high operative risk.

The following categories of patients are eligible for the prospective study: RO, patients without myometrial invasion, any G; RE, patients with pathologic stage II (occult involvement of the cervix), stage III (involvement of ovaries, free tract of fallopian tubes, pelvic peritoneum, parametrium), stage IV A (involvement beyond the true pelvis).

The RO and RE categories are submitted to follow-up like the valid cases.

The risk categories eligible for the study are randomized, either to receive or not adjuvant hormone treatment with MPA, 100 mg twice a day by mouth for 12 months. The treatment plan is the following: R1, surgery alone versus surgery plus MPA; R2, surgery plus radiotherapy on the pelvis (50 Gy in 5–7 weeks) versus the same plus MPA; R3, surgery plus radiotherapy on the pelvis as in R2 plus para-aortic chains (45 Gy in 5–7 weeks plus boost with 10 Gy on involved lymph nodes) versus the same plus MPA.

FOLLOW-UP

The patients are submitted to follow-up (clinical and pelvic examination) every 2 months in the first year, every 3 months in the second year, every 4 months i., the third year, and then every 6 and 12 months in the 2 subsequent years, respectively. Chest X-ray, X-ray of the pelvic bone, vaginal smear, and blood chemistry should be performed every 6 months in the first year and then every 12 months. Intravenous urography should be performed 1 month after surgery and with barium enema 6 months after radiotherapy.

REGISTERED PATIENTS AND VALID PATIENTS

The protocol study was activated in February 1980 and 21 Institutes are involved in the ongoing study. From February 1, 1980 to May 31, 1981 a total of 530 patients were registered: 116 were ineligible and 414 eligible for the study. There were 18 protocol violations. Three hundred and ninety-six patients are evaluable and 270 (R1 = 144, R2 = 120, R3 = 6) were randomized (Table 3).

The majority of patients had an age between 51 and 60 years. The distribution of patients according to histology and the comparison between curettage and surgical specimen are reported in Table 4. The majority of the patients (81.1%) had an adenocarcinoma and the minority a clear-cell carcinoma (0.7%). The comparison between curettage and surgical specimen showed many patients (33 patients) with a change of histologic diagnosis. The histopathologic grade was 1 in 55.9%, grade 2 in 31.9%, and grade 3 in 11.1%. Information is still not available for three cases (Table 5).

LYMPHOGRAPHY IN THE STUDY PROTOCOL

For the diagnosis of metastatic involvement the criteria described by Piver et al. (37), Douglas et al. (14), Wallace et al. (44), and Musumeci et al. (30) will be used. At the time of this writing the lymphangiograms have yet to be reinterpreted by the consultant radiologists.

Of the 270 valid cases, lymphography was negative in 206 patients and positive in nine. In 41 patients the lymphangiograms were doubtful and in 14 patients

TABLE 3. *Controlled clinical study on stage I endometrial carcinoma—CNR 07179/N*

Registered patients and valid patients		Totals
Registered cases		530
Ineligible cases		116
age > 75 yrs		17
refuse diagnostic work-up		1
previous neoplastic disease		11
synchronous neoplastic disease		8
previous treatment		1
mixed mesodermal tumors		5
exitus presurgery		1
no surgery for high operative risk (RX)		10
vaginal hysterectomy for high operative risk (RV)		16
geographic inaccessibility		5
severe disease		4
exitus postsurgery		2
radiotherapy not feasible		3
incomplete radiologic work-up		5
incomplete surgical staging (± radiologic work-up)		4
others		2
multiple		21
Considered eligible cases		414
Evaluable cases		396
patients evaluable only for natural history		126
RO:	66	
RE:	60	
Patients in controlled study		270
R1: 144 ⟋ MPA:	69	
⟍ NO MPA:	75	
R2: 120 ⟋ MPA:	61	
⟍ NO MPA:	59	
R3: 6 ⟋ MPA:	2	
⟍ NO MPA:	4	
Protocol violations (error in eligibility)		18/414 (4.3%)
cases evaluable only for natural history		0/126
cases eligible for randomized study		18/288 (6.2%)

TABLE 4. *Controlled clinical trial on stage I endometrial carcinoma—CNR 07179/N[a]*

Curettage	Surgical specimen	Adeno-carcinoma	Adeno-acanthoma	Clear cell carcinoma	Adenosquamous carcinoma	Undifferen-tiated	Missing Information
Adenocarcinoma	222	199	12	—	8	2	1
Adenoacanthoma	17	4	11	—	2	—	—
Clear cell carcinoma	1	—	—	1	—	—	—
Adenosquamous carcinoma	7	—	1	—	6	—	—
Squamous carcinoma	1	—	—	1	1	—	—
Undifferentiated carcinoma	3	—	—	—	—	2	—
Atypical hyperplasia	2	2	—	—	—	—	—
Missing information	17	14	1	—	1	—	1
Total	270	219 81.1	25 9.3	2 0.7	18 6.7	4 1.5	2 0.7

[a]Histology: comparison between curettage and surgical specimen.

TABLE 5. *Controlled clinical trial on stage I endometrial carcinoma—*
CNR 07179/N[a]

		G1	G2	G3	Missing information
Adenocarcinoma	219	134	66	17	2
		61.0	30.3	7.8	0.9
Adenoacanthoma	25	11	12	2	—
		44.0	48.0	8.0	
Clear cell	2	1	—	1	—
carcinoma		50.0		50.0	
Adenosquamous	18	4	8	5	1
carcinoma		23.5	41.2	29.4	5.9
Undifferentiated	4	—	—	4	—
carcinoma				100.0	
Missing	2	1	—	1	—
information		50.0		50.0	
Total	270	151	86	30	3
		55.9	31.9	11.1	1.1

[a]Histopathological grading—patients in controlled study: 270.

equivocal. Retroperitoneal node biopsies were performed in a total of 133 of 270 valid cases. Histology of retroperitoneal nodes was negative in 127 patients and positive in 6 patients. The histologic-radiologic correlation showed a large percentage of false-positive and false-negative cases at lymphography.

PATHOLOGIC STAGE IN THE STUDY PROTOCOL

Of 396 evaluable patients submitted to total abdominal hysterectomy plus bilateral salpingo-oophorectomy plus colpectomy of the superior third of the vagina plus selective or systematic pelvic and/or para-aortic node biopsies, 329 remained stage IA-IB (83%).

Forty-five patients were definitively classified as stage II, 43 for endocervical and two for ectocervical extension. Twenty-one patients were definitively classified as stage III and one as stage IV for omental involvement. In the group of patients classified as stage III there were 6 cases randomized in the R3 risk group (primary tumor limited to the uterus with histological retroperitoneal node involvement). The single conversion rate was 11.4% from stage I to stage II, 5.3% from stage I to stage III, and 0.2% from stage I to stage IV (Table 6).

Protocol treatment is regularly performed in all patients.

No patient has been lost to follow-up. No other data are presently available for this study. The study allows the entry of patients until December 1983. It should be possible to evaluate a large number of cases in a prospective manner for the natural history, spread of disease, and randomized treatment.

ACKNOWLEDGMENT

This study was performed by the Subproject "Clinical Multimodality Therapy" of the Applications-Oriented Project "Control of Neoplastic Growth" of the National Research Council of Italy.

TABLE 6. *Controlled clinical study on stage I endometrial carcinoma—CNR 07179/N*

Cases FIGO stage I submitted to surgery[a]	→396	%
Pathological stage:		
IA–IB→	329	(83)
II→	45	(11.4)
III→	21[b]	(5.3)
IVA→	1	(0.25)

[a]TAH + BSO + colpectomy plus selective or systematic retroperitoneal node biopsies.
[b]Six cases were randomized in the R3 risk group (primary tumor limited at the uterus with regional lymph node involvement).

Participating Institutions were: I Department of Obstetrics and Gynecology, University of Milano (Responsible Investigator: C. Mangioni, M.D.); II Department of Obstetrics and Gynecology, University of Milano (Responsible Investigator: F. Acerboni, M.D.); V Department of Obstetrics and Gynecology, University of Milano (Responsible Investigator: M. Vignali, M.D.); Department of Obstetrics and Gynecology "Macedonio Melloni" of Milano (Responsible Investigator: E. Saraceno, M.D.); I Department of Obstetrics and Gynecology, University of Bari (Responsible Investigator: S. Bettocchi, M.D.); II Department of Obstetrics and Gynecology, University of Bari (Responsible Investigator: G. Cagnazzo, M.D.); I Department of Obstetrics and Gynecology, University of Bologna (Responsible Investigator: G. Sani, M.D.); II Department of Obstetrics and Gynecology, University of Bologna (Responsible Investigator: C. Orlandi, M.D.); III Department of Obstetrics and Gynecology, University of Milano (Responsible Investigator: U. Bianchi, M.D.); Department of Obstetrics and Gynecology, University of Catania (Responsible Investigator: S. Di Leo, M.D.); Department of Obstetrics and Gynecology, University of Firenze (Responsible Investigator: F. Gasparri, M.D.); Department of Obstetrics and Gynecology, University of Genova (Responsible Investigator: F. Pescetto, M.D.); Department of Obstetrics and Gynecology, University of Padova (Responsible Investigator: A. Onnis, M.D.); Department of Obstetrics and Gynecology, University of Pavia (Responsible Investigator: V. Danesino, M.D.); Department of Obstetrics and Gynecology, University of Pisa (Responsible Investigator: P. Fioretti, M.D.); I Department of Obstetrics and Gynecology, University of Torino (Responsible Investigator: P. Sismondi, M.D.); II Department of Obstetrics and Gynecology, University of Torino (Responsible Investigator: R. Monti, M.D.); II Department of Obstetrics and Gynecology, University of Roma (Responsible Investigator: L. Carenza, M.D.); Department of Oncologic Gynecology, Cancer Institute of Roma (Responsible Investigator: P. Marziale, M.D.); Department of Obstetrics and Gynecology, University of "Sacro Cuore" of Roma (Responsible Investigator: S. Dell'Acqua, M.D.); Department of Obstetrics and Gynecology, University of Ferrara (Responsible Investigator: G. Mollica, M.D.). Statistician Group of Subproject "Combined Therapies," National Cancer Institute of Milano: E. Marubini, G. Gallus, M. Del Vecchio, P. Valagussa.

REFERENCES

1. Aalders, J., Abeler, V., Kolstad, P., and Onsrud, M. (1980): *Obstet. Gynecol.*, 56:419.
2. Berman, M. L., and Ballon, S. C. (1979): *Cancer Treat. Rev.*, 6:165.
3. Bonte, J., Decoster, J. M., and Ide, P. (1970): *Cancer*, 25:907.
4. Bonte, J., Decoster, J. M., Ide, P., Wynants, P., and Billiet, G. (1974): In: *Recent Progress in Obstetrics and Gynaecology*, pp. 205–297. Excerpta Medica Amsterdam; Avicenum Czeckoslovak Medical Press, Prague.
5. Boyd, I. E., Pollard, W., and Blaikley, J. B. (1973): *J. Obstet. Gynaecol. Br. Commonw.*, 80:360.
6. Brady, L. W. (1975): *Cancer*, 35:76.
7. Cheon, H. K. (1969): *Obstet. Gynecol.*, 34:680.
8. Creasman, W. T., Boronow, R. C., Morrow, P. C., Di Saia, P. J., and Blessing, J. (1976): *Gynecol. Oncol.*, 4:239.
9. Creasman, W. T., and Rutledge, F. N. (1971): *Am. J. Obstet. Gynecol.*, 110:773.
10. De Palo, G., Bandieramonte, G., Kenda, R., et al. (1978): *Attl. Soc. It. Ost. Gin.*, 59:481.
11. De Palo, G., Kenda, R., Andreola, S., Luciani, L., Muscumeci, R., and Rilke, F.: Endometrial carcinoma: pathologic stage I. A retrospective analysis of 262 patients. *In press.*
12. De Palo, G., Kenda, R., Bandieramonte, G., De Menech, D., and Muscumeci, R. (1979): *Obstet. Ginecol. Lat. Am.*, 37:121.
13. Di Saia, P. I., and Creasman, W. T. (1981): *Clinical Gynecologic Oncology*, Mosby, St. Louis, Toronto, London.
14. Douglas, B., Macdonald, J. S., and Baker, J. W. (1972): *Clin. Radiol.*, 23:286.
15. Fuchs, W. A. (1969): In: *Lymphography in Cancer: Recent Results in Cancer Research*, edited by W. A. Fuchs, J. W. Davidson, and H. W. Fisher, p. 116. Springer Verlag, Berlin, Heidelberg, New York.
16. Gerteis, W. (1967): In: Ruttiman, A., ed. *Progress in Lymphology*, edited by A. Ruttiman, p. 209. George Thieme Verlag, Stuttgart.
17. Hawksworth, W. (1964): *Proc. Roy. Soc. Med.*, 57:467.
18. Henriksen, E. (1949): *Am. J. Obstet. Gynecol.*, 58:924.
19. Homesley, H. D., Boronow, R. C., and Lewis, J. L. (1977): *Obstet. Gynecol.*, 49:604.
20. Jones, H. W. (1975): *Obstet. Gynecol. Surv.*, 30:147.
21. Kademian, M. T., Buchler, T. A., and Wirtanen, G. W. (1977): *Am. J. Roentgenol.*, 129:903.
22. Lees, D. H. (1969): *J. Obstet. Gynaecol. Br. Commonw.*, 76:615.
23. Lewis, B. U., Stallworthy, J. A., and Cowdell, R. (1970): *J. Obstet. Gynaecol. Br. Commonw.*, 77:343.
24. Lewis, G. C., Jr., Slack, N. H., Mortel, R., and Bross, I. D. J. (1974): *Gynec. Oncol.*, 2:368.
25. Liu, W., and Meigs, J. V. (1955): *Am. J. Obstet. Gynecol.*, 69:1.
26. Lutz, M. H., Underwood, P. B., Jr., Kreutner, A., Jr., and Miller, M. (1978): *Gynecol. Oncol.*, 6:83.
27. Malkasian, G. D. (1978): *Cancer*, 41:996.
28. Malkasian, G. D., Annegers, J. F., and Fountain, K. S. (1980): *Am. J. Obstet. Gynecol.*, 136:872.
29. Morrow, C. P., Di Saia, P. J., and Townsend, D. E. (1973): *Obstet. Gynecol.*, 42:399.
30. Musumeci, R., Banfi, A., Bolis, G., Candiani, G. B., De Palo, G., Di Re, F., Luciani, L., Lattuada, A., Mangioni, C., Mattioli, G., and Natale, N. (1977): *Cancer*, 40:1444.
31. Musumeci, R., De Palo, G., Conti, U., Kenda, R., Mangioni, C., Belloni, C., Marzi, M., and Bandieramonte, G. (1980): *Cancer*, 46:1887.
32. Musumeci, R., Kenda, R., Volterrani, F., Spatti, G. B., Luciani, L., Attili, A., and De Palo, G. (1979): *Tumori*, 65:77.
33. Ng, A. B., and Reagan, J. W. (1970): *Obstet. Gynecol.*, 35:437.
34. Nolan, J. F., and Huen, H. (1976): *Gynec. Oncol.*, 4:384.
35. Nolan, J. F., Morrow, C. P., and Anson, J. (1974): *Gynec. Oncol.*, 2:300.
36. Periti, P., and Mini, E. (1978): In: *Le Neoplasie dell'Apparato Genitale Femminile*. CEA Ed., Milano.
37. Piver, M. S., Wallace, S., and Castro, R. 1971): *Am. J. Roentgenol.*, 111:278.
38. Plentl, A. A., and Friedman, E. A. (1971): *Lymphatic System of the Female Genitalia*. Saunders, Philadelphia.
39. Rouviere, H. (1932): *Anatomie des lymphatiques de l'homme*. Masson et Cie, Paris.
40. Rickford, R. B. K. (1968): *J. Obstet. Gynaecol. Br. Commonw.*, 75:580.
41. Roberts, D. W. T. (1961): *J. Obstet. Gynaecol. Br. Commonw.*, 68:132.

42. Salazar, O. M., Feldstein, M. L., De Papp, E. W., Bonfiglio, T. A., Keller, B. E., Rubin, P., and Rudolph, J. H. (1978): *Cancer*, 41:1016.
43. Schwartz, A. E., and Brunschwing, A. (1957): *Surg. Gynecol. Obstet.*, 105:675.
44. Wallace, S., Jing, B., and Medellin, H. (1974): *Gynecol. Obstet.*, 2:287.

Role of Medroxyprogesterone in Endocrine-Related Tumors, Volume II, edited by L. Campio, G. Robustelli Della Cuna, and R. W. Taylor. Raven Press, New York © 1983.

The Treatment of Ovarian Cancer with Medroxyprogesterone Acetate

C. Bumma, O. Bertetto, and *G. Gentile

*Department of Oncology, S. Giovanni Battista Hospital, 10100 Turin; *Ospedale Civile, 14100 Asti, Italy*

The determination of hormonal receptors is currently a valid method for the clinical evaluation of endocrine-related breast and endometrial cancer and is helpful in the choice of treatment. Obviously, tumors with high level of receptors have a higher response to endocrine therapy (11). In our preliminary research (1,2), we found, in epithelial ovarian carcinoma, progesterone and estrogen receptors in only 25% of the cases (total: 32 patients) (Table 1).

The natural history of epithelial ovarian carcinoma suggests that it may have a hormonal etiology just as breast cancer and endometrial carcinoma; unfortunately the results obtained with hormonal treatment have been rather poor, perhaps because it has been used in poorly selected patients (7,8). In describing the results of personal research, D. H. Darwish (3) reports on 12 ovarian tumors studied by means of short organ tissue culture: He observed the effects of different sex steroids on the *in vitro* DNA synthesis and reported that 17-beta-estradiol, in combination with progesterone, reduced the DNA synthesis by 60–80% and that progesterone alone gave a reduction of 50–75%. However due to the rapid progression of ovarian carcinoma,

TABLE 1. *Hormonal receptors in ovarian carcinoma*

Pt. No.	Site	Histology	Receptors[a] (Fmoles/mg prot.)	
			ER	PgR
1	Peritoneum	Epithelial	14	5
2	Ovary	Epithelial	33	9
3	Ovary	Adenocarcinoma	19	7
4	Ovary	Epithelial	5	9
5	Peritoneum	Adenocarcinoma	12	5
6	Peritoneum	Adenocarcinoma	5	10
7	Ovary	Epithelial	19	9
8	Ovary	Epithelial	0	9

[a]The receptors were detected in 32 patients. Receptor-positive 8/32 (25%). ER, estrogen receptor; PgR, progesterone receptor.

there is a need for rapidly acting chemotherapeutic agents. The combination of chemotherapy with hormonotherapy seems of particular interest since with this therapeutic approach higher response rates could be achieved (13).

This study reports the results obtained in a group of patients affected by ovarian carcinoma and treated with a combination of chemotherapy and endocrine therapy. The comparison of the results has been done with a group of patients treated with chemotherapy lone. The object of the study was to evaluate the increase of cytotoxic effect obtained with the combination chemohormono treatment.

MATERIALS AND METHODS

Between 1977 and 1979, 50 patients suffering from epithelial ovarian carcinoma entered into the study. Out of 50 patients, 42 could be evaluated, 6 were lost at follow-up, and 2 died during the treatment. Table 2 reports the clinical characteristics of these patients.

Before entering into the study all patients were carefully examined with an accurate staging of the disease as well as diagnosis confirmed by histology, and recording of any information related to previous treatment. The patients were randomly (closed-envelope system) assigned to one of the two groups of treatment to receive either chemotherapy (FAC) or chemotherapy plus medroxyprogesterone acetate (MPA), according to the following scheme:

TABLE 2. *Clinical characteristics of patients included in the study*

		Treatment	
		FAC	FAC + MPA
Patients enrolled	(no.)	25	25
Patients evaluable	(no.)	19	22
Median age	(yr.)	53	55
Stage III	(no.)	9	9
Stage IV	(no.)	16	16

TABLE 3. *Results obtained in stage III patients*

		Treatment	
		FAC	FAC + MPA
Patients enrolled	(no.)	12	12
Patients evaluable	(no.)	10	11
CR (confirmed by laparoscopy)	(no.)	2 (20%)	3 (27%)
PR (confirmed by laparoscopy)	(no.)	5 (50%)	6 (54%)
CR + PR	(%)	70	81
Duration of response (median)	(months)	11	18

Group A: Chemotherapy (FAC)
   Fluorouracil: 500 mg/m^2 i.v., day 1 and 8
   Adriamycin: 30 mg/m^2 i.v., day 1 and 8
   Cyclophosphamide: 100 mg/m^2 p.o., day 1 to 14
followed by 14 days without treatment.

Group B: Chemotherapy (FAC) as above *plus*
   MPA: 500 mg i.m. for 30 days, then twice a week

This regimen was administered for a total of 6 courses up to a total dose of adriamycin of 400 mg/m^2. The results were evaluated every fourth week by means of physical and laboratory examinations. All patients were carefully reevaluated after 6 months of treatment. The follow-up procedure included physical examination, chest X-ray, skeletal survey, TAC, second-look laparascopy and/or laparotomy.

RESULTS

The evaluation of therapeutic response was done according to the criteria listed below:

Complete remission (CR): disappearance of all known lesions, documented in
   ovarian carcinoma by second-look laparoscopy and/or laparotomy;
Partial remission (PR): a 50% decrease in measurable lesions;
No change (NC): lesions are unchanged;
Progressive disease (P): some lesions progress or new lesions appear.

The duration of remission was recorded from the starting of the treatment.

Table 3 reports the results obtained in patients with disease in stage III. It should be noted that CR (confirmed by laparoscopy) was achieved in 2 patients treated with chemotherapy alone and in 3 patients treated with chemotherapy plus MPA. The percentage of PR was similar in both groups; however, patients treated with the association of chemo- and hormonotherapy achieved a longer duration of response than those treated with chemotherapy alone.

TABLE 4. *Results obtained in stage IV patients*

		Treatment	
		FAC	FAC + MPA
Patients enrolled	(no.)	13	13
Patients evaluable	(no.)	9	12
CR	(no.)	0	0
PR	(no.)	5 (55%)	8 (66%)
Duration of response (median)	(months)	7	13

TABLE 5. *Side effects*

	Treatment	
	FAC	FAC + MPA
Hair loss	12/19 (68%)	13/21 (61%)
Cardiotoxicity (+)	2/19 (10%)	3/21 (14%)
Moon faces	0/19	2/21 (9.5%)
Vaginal bleeding	0/19	3/21 (14%)
Gluteal abscess	0/19	3/21 (14%)
Increase of arterial pressure	1/19 (0.5%)	3/21 (14%)
Increase of body weight	0/19	13/21 (61%)
Strong myelosuppression	50%	20%

(+) ECK abnormality: RS-T depression, inversion of T wave.

Also patients in stage IV of the disease had a longer duration of response if treated with chemotherapy associated with MPA (Table 4). Side effects related to the treatment are reported in Table 5; gluteal abscess, moon faces, and considerable anabolizing activity are reported only in the group of patients receiving hormonal therapy; hematological toxicity (leukopenia <2000 leukocytes/mm^3 and thrombocytopenia $<60,000$ platelets/mm^3) was more severe in the group of patients receiving chemotherapy alone. This confirms data already reported and clarified by other investigators (13).

CONCLUSIONS

On the basis of our experience the combination of hormone plus chemotherapy appears encouraging, with response rates similar to those obtained with chemotherapy alone and with a longer duration of the median response. Endocrine therapy may therefore stabilize the therapeutic results of chemotherapy.

The "quality of life" of the patients treated with FAC + MPA was better than that obtained with chemotherapy alone. Lowering the toxic effect at bone marrow level with the inclusion of MPA in the chemotherapy scheme and obtaining the remission of some symptoms such as anorexia and asthenia thus made it possible in some instances to prolong the administration of chemotherapeutic agents. It is also our opinion that better results with hormonal treatment can be achieved in cases of ovarian cancer selected on the basis of hormonal receptors.

REFERENCES

1. Bumma, C., and Castronuovo, G. (1979): *Boll. Soc. Piemontese di Chirurgia*, 3:367–372.
2. Calciati, A., Bumma, C., Serra, M. C., and Di Carlo, F. (1979): *Riunioni Integrate di Oncologia*, Ancona May 26–28 *(Abstr.)*, p. 75.
3. Darwish, D. H. (1978): *Br. J. Obstet. Gynecol.*, 85:627–633.
4. Davy, M., Torjesan, P. A., and Aakvaag, A. (1977): *Acta Endocrinol.*, 85:615–623.
5. De Lena, M., Brambilla, C., Morabito, A., and Bonadonna, G. (1975): *Cancer*, 35:1108–1115.
6. Friberg, L. G. (1978): *Acta Obstet. Gynecol. Scand.*, 57:261–264.
7. Kammerman, S., and Ross, J. (1975): *J. Clin. Endocrinol. Metab.*, 41:546–550.
8. Kammerman, S., Demopulos, R., and Ross, J. (1977): *Cancer Res.*, 37:2578–82.

9. Kiang, D. T., and Kennedy, B. J. (1977): *J. Am. Med. Assoc.*, 238:32–34.
10. Lee, C. Y., and Ryan, R. Y. (1973): In: *Receptors for Reproductive Hormones*, pp. 410–429. Plenum Press, New York.
11. McGuire, W. L. (1975): *Cancer*, 36:638–650.
12. Pannuti, F., Martoni, A., Di Marco, A. R., Piana, E., and Nanni, P. (1978): *Cancer Treatment Rep.*, 62:499–504.
13. Robustelli Della Cuna, G., and Bernardo Strada, M. R. (1980): In: *Role of Medroxyprogesterone in Endocrine-Related Tumors*, edited by S. Iacobelli and A. Di Marco, pp. 53–65. Raven Press, New York.

Role of Medroxyprogesterone in Endocrine-Related Tumors, Volume II, edited by L. Campio, G. Robustelli Della Cuna, and R. W. Taylor. Raven Press, New York © 1983.

Medroxyprogesterone Acetate in the Treatment of Prostatic Cancer: Preliminary Results of EORTC Trial 30761 Comparing MPA with Stilbestrol and with Cyproterone Acetate

M. Pavone-Macaluso and the EORTC Urological Group

*EORTC Urological Group and Department of Urology, Polyclinic Hospital, University of Palermo School of Medicine, 90127 Palermo, Italy; *EORTC Data Center, Brussels, Belgium*

New treatment modalities are currently under investigation as an alternative to conventional estrogenic therapy in advanced prostatic cancer, especially as the cardiovascular toxicity of high doses of estrogens has been clearly elucidated.

The value of and the indications for orchidectomy and hormonal treatment of prostatic cancer still remain controversial. To our present knowledge it is impossible to establish any fast rule as to the best treatment to be adopted in the various stages of the disease, and especially in some situations such as poorly differentiated carcinoma and cancer which is unresponsive to hormonal treatment, due either to primary resistance or to secondary relapse (4).

Although hormonal therapy still remains an effective form of treatment, the initial enthusiasm was decreased by the discovery of the cardiovascular side effects of estrogens. It is well known that hormonal treatment does not lead to a permanent cure. Objective regression can be demonstrated in less than one-half of cases. Therefore, hormonal treatment is basically a palliative measure which may have a rather prolonged duration and may lead to stabilization in relatively large number of cases.

*EORTC Data Center, Brussels, Belgium: M. De Pauw, S. Suciu, R. Sylvester. Participants in protocols 30761 and 30762: *United Kingdom*: P. H. Smith, J. R. G. Bastable, R. Glashan, D. Newling, B. Richards, M. R. G. Robinson, R. E. Williams; *Italy*: M. Pavone-Macaluso, C. Bondavalli, G. Castaldi, M. Laudi, S. Leoni, F. Merlo, V. Nadalini, A. Nasta, M. Porena, C. Viggiano, E. Visentini, R. Zolfanelli; *The Netherlands*: H. De Voogt, J. Alexieva; *France*: B. Lardennois, J. Guerrin; *Belgium*: C. Bouffioux, C. Schulman; *Spain*: J. A. Martinez-Pineiro, E. A. Barrilero, L. Resell-Esteve; *Portugal*: F. Calais da Silva; *Austria*: J. Frick.

There is obviously a need for investigating new modalities of hormonal treatment for prostatic cancer in the hope to discover new forms of therapy displaying a higher efficacy and a lower incidence of side effects. Unfortunately the majority of papers published on the topic of hormonal therapy are based on small series of patients, without control groups and with nonuniform response criteria.

The urological cooperative research group of the European Organization for Research on Treatment of Cancer (EORTC) has implemented a series of prospective, randomized clinical trials in recent years, hoping to give at least a few answers to some unsettled questions. Medroxyprogesterone acetate (MPA) was one of the arms of a trial (protocol 30761) that has been submitted to a preliminary analysis. This study was activated in February 1977 and closed to entry in April 1981. The results of the most recent analysis will be given here. Brief information will also be given on a parallel study conducted by the same cooperative group (protocol 30762) which compared diethylstilbestrol (DES) 3 mg versus estramustine phosphate (EMP), 560 mg p.d. orally for 8 weeks, 280 mg daily thereafter. (Study coordinator: P. H. Smith, Leeds.) Preliminary interim reports of both studies have already been published elsewhere (9,10).

PROTOCOL 30761

Purpose of the Study

The aim of this study (Study coordinator: M. Pavone-Macaluso, Palermo, Italy) was that of comparing DES, MPA, and cyproterone acetate (CPA) in a randomized trial, with regard to local and general objective response, duration of remission, toxicity, and survival in patients with advanced prostatic cancer.

Drugs Employed

A. DES is the conventional estrogenic treatment in USA, U.K., and some European countries. It is no longer commercially available in Italy.

B. MPA, like other progestational agents, inhibits LH release and decreases plasma testosterone levels and testosterone synthesis. As demonstrated by Massa and Martini (8), it also acts directly upon the prostatic tissue by inhibiting 5-alpha reductase and thereby reducing the formation of dihydrotestosterone (DHT) in normal and neoplastic prostatic cells.

A few pilot studies have demonstrated that MPA is active in prostatic cancer. Ferulano et al. (6) in 1972 described a few palliative and objective responses. In 1976 Belgian workers, namely Denis and Leclerq in Antwerp (5) and Bouffioux in Liège (1), reached similar results. An Italian cooperative study which we led in urological institutions in Palermo, Torino, and Cagliari (11) allowed us to observe that, of 62 evaluable patients, an objective response was obtained in 38.7% and a stabilization in another 37% of patients. It is of interest that responses were also obtained in patients who were relapsing after an initially favorable response to orchidectomy and/or estrogenic treatment.

In a controlled randomized trial (VACURG study III) (3), MPA 30 mg daily was not significantly inferior to DES, 1 mg/day. The results were not improved by combining DES and MPA.

C. CPA, apart from inhibition of LH release, acts through competitive inhibition of androgen receptors in target tissues. After the work reported by Bracci and Di Silverio (2) and Giuliani et al. (7), it has gained considerable popularity in Italy where it is usually employed in conjunction with orchidectomy, but has not yet been introduced in the United States as an accepted treatment for prostatic cancer.

Admission Criteria

Only patients not having been submitted to previous hormonal treatment or orchidectomy were eligible for this study. All patients had histologically confirmed and locally advanced prostatic carcinoma (categories T3 and T4), with or without distant metastases. Patients with a life expectancy below 90 days and those with severe cardiovascular disease contraindicating estrogenic treatment were not admitted to the study.

Doses and Modalities of Administration of the Hormonal Compounds

After randomization, one of the following treatments was started: (a) DES—3 mg daily (1 mg every 8 hr, orally); (b) MPA—loading dose: 500 mg i.m. 3 times weekly for 8 weeks; maintenance dose: 100 mg twice daily, per os; (c) CPA—250 mg daily, per os.

The first control visit was performed at 2 months from start of therapy. If at the second visit, i.e., at 4 months, progression was evident, the patient was put off study. In the case of response, the treatment was continued and in the case of stable disease, the investigators were left free to continue or to modify the original treatment. It occurred, however, that almost all patients with stabilization were maintained on the initial treatment.

Response Criteria

Objective responses were classified as CR (complete regression), PR (partial regression), NC (no change) or PD (progressive disease). The response of the primary tumor was assessed by digital rectal palpation. The response criteria were as follows: CR, absence of palpable neoplastic mass or induration; PR, local regression greater than 50% of the product of the two largest diameters; NC, objective changes less than 50%; PD, increase of local mass greater than 50%.

Similar criteria were adopted for the osseous metastases. The details are given in the original protocols. All X-rays and bone scans were reviewed by an extramural review committee, having no knowledge of the treatment given to the individual patients. To fulfill the criteria for CR, a normalization of serum acid phosphatase (SAP) was requested, if previously elevated. Conversely, an *isolated* increase of SAP was not judged as a certain sign of progression. Stabilization of disease was not classified as a therapeutic response.

Preliminary Results

The preliminary results were assessed for toxicity and cumulative objective response. The 295 patients who entered the study were evenly distributed in the 3 treatment groups.

Patients were entered from several urological institutions from Italy, U.K., Belgium, the Netherlands, France, Spain, Portugal, and Austria. About one-half of the patients were treated in urological centers in Italy, as opposed to protocol 30762, where most patients were treated in U.K. (Table 1). The percentage of patients who were put off study for progression or death is not significantly different among the various treatment groups (Table 2). With regard to side effects, painful gynecomastia were more frequent in patients treated with DES than with either MPA or CPA (Table 3). Gastrointestinal side effects were more frequent in patients given EMP than in those receiving MPA, DES, or CPA (Table 4).

Concerning cardiovascular (CV) toxicity (Table 5) the total number of CV complications is less in the CPA group than in DES or MPA groups. This difference

TABLE 1. *Geographical distribution of patients*

Country	Prot. 30761	Prot. 30762
Italy	146 (49%)	—
The Netherlands	52	—
France	38	10
United Kingdom	28	220 (90%)
Spain	17	—
Belgium	7	15
Portugal	5	—
Austria	2	—
Total	295	248

TABLE 2. *Reasons for going off study*

	Prot. 30761			Prot. 30762	
	DES	MPA	CPA	DES	FEM
1. Progression (including cancer death)	44	52	43	36	49
2. Death related to other causes	7.5	3	6	21	10
3. Excessive toxicity	4	4.5	2	14	19
4. Treatment refused	5.5	7.5	10	6	5
5. Loss on follow-up	11	12	26	3	0
6. Protocol violations (including eligibility criteria)	13	15	8	17	10
7. Other causes	15	6	5	3	7

Figures represent percentage values.

TABLE 3. *Painful gynecomastia by treatment groups*

Treatment	No. of pts.	Painful gynecomastia present
DES	52	21 (40%)
MAP	52	3 (6%)
CPA	52	3 (6%)
Total	156	27 (17%)

TABLE 4. *Gastrointestinal side effects by treatment groups*

	Prot. 30761			Prot. 30762	
	DES	MPA	CPA	DES	FEM
No changes in treatment	0 (0)	3 (6)	1 (2)	9 (9)	13 (17)
Brief interruption or change in treatment	1 (2)	1 (2)	0 (0)	2 (2)	4 (5)
Termination of treatment	0 (0)	0 (0)	0 (0)	0 (0)	8 (11)
Total number of patients with GI symptoms	1 (2)	4 (8)	1 (2)	11 (11)	25 (33)
Total number of treated patients	52	52	52	101	75

Percentages are given in parentheses.

TABLE 5. *Cardiovascular side effects*

	Prot. 30761			Prot. 30762	
	DES	MPA	CPA	DES	FEM
Mild	18 (31)	9 (14)	4 (7)	19 (18)	18 (17)
Moderate (termination of treatment)	2 (3.5)	3 (5)	0 (0)	9 (8)	8 (7)
Lethal	2 (3.5)	1 (1)	4 (7)	10 (9)	3 (3)
Total number of patients with CV side effects	22 (38)	13 (20)	8 (14)	38 (35)	29 (27)
Total number of treated patients	58	64	57	107	107

Percentages are given in parentheses.

is statistically significant. It should be noted, however, that the percentage of lethal CV complications was higher in CPA-treated patients than in the other groups (CPA, 7%; DES, 3.5%; MPA, 1%). Regarding DES, the number and severity of CV complications were higher in the Anglo-Saxon (protocol 30762) than in the Italian or other Latin patients (protocol 30761). It should be stressed that none of the treatment modalities under investigation was devoid of some CV toxicity, although its severity and incidence rate were not identical in the various groups.

The CV toxicity was classified under one of the following headings: ischemic cardiopathy; thromboembolic complications; fluid retention (Table 6). The severe complications were present in all of these categories. No significant difference in this distribution was observed in relation to the treatment. As far as the incidence of CV disease prior to the treatment is concerned, some interesting observations can be made (Table 7). In patients with a previous history of CV disease, MPA was associated with the lowest incidence of CV complications. Conversely, in patients without CV disease before the treatment, CPA appeared to be best tolerated. The difference between DES and CPA is significant in this respect.

Local and distant objective responses were analyzed together for protocol 30761 (Table 8). All the three hormonal compounds produced objective responses (CR + PR: 44% for DES; 33% for CPA and 18% for MPA). No CR were observed in the MPA group. The following p values were calculated: MPA vs DES: $p = 0.005$; CPA vs DES: $p = 0.32$; CPA vs MPA: $p = 0.12$. It appears therefore that only the difference between DES and MPA is statistically significant.

Study 30762 showed that DES is somewhat superior to Estracyt® ($p = 0.13$) with regard to the response of the primary lesion, whereas both treatments appear

TABLE 6. *Type of cardiovascular complications*

	Prot. 30761			Prot. 30762			
	DES	MPA	CPA	DES	FEM	Total[a]	Lethal cases
Ischemic cardiopathy	10.5	6	3.5	9	4	7	2
Thromboembolic diseases	10.5	6	3.5	8	7	7	2
Fluid retention	17	6	7	18	15	13	4
Not specified	0	2	0	0	1	0	0
Total	38	20	14	35	27	27	8

Figures represent percentage values.
[a]For both protocols, from a total number of 393 patients.

TABLE 7. *Percentage of patients with CV side effects, related to the presence or absence of CV symptoms at the beginning of therapy*

Previous CV symptoms	Prot. 30761				Prot. 30762		
	DES	MPA	CPA	Total	DES	FEM	Total
Yes	48	19	29	31	52	26	37
No	32[b]	26	8[b]	22	32	29	30
Total	38[a]	23	14[a]	25	36	28	32

DES vs CPA: [a]$p = 0.01$; [b]$p = 0.02$. The other differences are not statistically significant.

TABLE 8. *Protocol 30761: Cumulative objective responses (prostate and distant metastases) by treatment*

Treatment	No. of pts	CR	PR	NC	PD	% CR + PR
DES	57	7	18	18	14	44
MPA	56	0	10	23	23	18
CPA	52	2	15	14	21	33
Total	165	9	43	55	58	32

DES vs MPA, $p = 0.005$; DES vs CPA, $p = 0.32$; CPA vs MPA, $p = 0.12$.

equally effective upon the bone metastases, with a response rate of 30%. A few cases of complete disappearance of the hot spots on the bone scans were observed in both groups. The survival rates are better for DES than for EMP in spite of the higher CV toxicity due to the estrogen. The final analyses of both protocols are awaited with the greatest interest.

CONCLUSIONS

In previously untreated patients with advanced prostatic cancer, DES appears to remain, at least, no worse than the newest hormonal compounds. It is certainly cheaper and it shows a statistically significant superiority over MPA. It should be stressed, however, that DES, 3 mg/day, is not devoid of CV toxicity, especially in Anglo-Saxon patients. MPA, whose palliative effects have been confirmed (though the data have not yet been given in detail) may represent a good alternative in symptomatic patients presenting a positive history of CV disease.

The present data of the EORTC urological group appear to indicate, therefore, that MPA does not represent the treatment to be employed as a first choice for the majority of patients with previously untreated adenocarcinoma of the prostate, at least at the dosage employed in this trial. However our own pilot studies, as well as those of other investigators, indicated that MPA may be of value in inducing a response in about one-third of the patients who are in relapse after an initial response to estrogens. As the symptomatic improvement is often dramatic, MPA is probably the treatment of choice in relapsing patients with well- or moderately differentiated adenocarcinoma of the prostate. Estracyt® or cytotoxic chemotherapy should be considered, on the other hand, in the relapsing patient with the poorly differentiated lesions. Very little is known about the value of the combination of MPA with chemotherapeutic agents in the treatment of prostatic cancer. This represents a very appealing avenue for further investigation in the near future. CPA does not appear to be superior to DES in the previously untreated patients, but it also shows activity and its low incidence of CV side effects deserves to be pointed out. Its value in association with orchidectomy or in combination with an antiprolactin drug will be evaluated in the two next trials activated by the EORTC urological group.

ADDENDUM

This paper was reviewed by the EORTC Data Center only after it had been submitted for publication. The Data Center felt that, from a statistical point of view, these two protocols are not strictly comparable due to the following differences:

1. The amount of available follow-up information is not uniform in the two protocols.
2. The response in protocol 30762 has been analyzed based on the review of scans and X-rays for the bone metastases on one hand, and the review of the primary tumor by The Data Center on the other hand. This is not the case for protocol 30761.
3. In protocol 30762, patients were left in the study as long as the investigators continued the assigned treatment, regardless as to whether or not they progressed, so that most of the patients were treated until death. In protocol 30761, however, the patients were taken off-study as soon as they progressed according to the local investigator. Therefore, the reasons for going off-study cannot be compared.

In preparing the final statistical analyses when both protocols will be nearer their final stage, it will be possible to eliminate these differences to a greater extent.

As these remarks are certainly appropriate, the readers should be warned, therefore, that any comparison between the two studies, as they appear in the text, should be merely considered as a possible trend or indication, pending the final analysis of both trials.

REFERENCES

1. Bouffioux, C. (1976): *Acta Urol. Belg.*, 44:336–353.
2. Bracci, U., and Di Silverio, F. (1979): In: *Terapia dei tumori ormonodipendenti*, edited by U. Bracci and F. Di Silverio, pp. 173–201, Acta Medica Ciarrapico, Rome.
3. Byar, D. (1977): In: *Tumours of Genito-Urinary Apparatus*, edited by M. Pavone-Macaluso, p. 275. Cofese, Palermo.
4. Chisholm, G. D., and Pavone-Macaluso, M. (1980): *Eur. Urol.*, 6:197–205.
5. Denis, L., and Leclercq, G. (1978): *Eur. Urol.*, 4:162–166.
6. Ferulano, O., Petrarola, F., and Castaldo, A. (1972): *Minerva Urol.*, 24:274–280.
7. Giuliani, L., Pescatore, D., Giberti, C., Martorana, G., and Natta, G. (1980): *Eur. Urol.*, 6:145–148.
8. Massa, R., and Martini, L. (1971–72): *Gynecol. Invest.*, 2:253–270.
9. Pavone-Macaluso, M., and EORTC Urological Group (1981): In: *Antihormone. Bedeutung in der Urologie*, edited by J. E. Altwein, G. Bartsch, and G. H. Jacobi, pp. 235–242. W. Zuckschwerdt Verlag, Munich.
10. Pavone-Macaluso, M., Lund, F., Mulder, J. H., Smith, P. H., De Pauw, M., Sylvester, R., and EORTC Urological Group (1980): *Scand. J. Urol. Nephrol.*, 55:163–168.
11. Pavone-Macaluso, M., Melloni, D., La Piana, E., Usai, E., Oggiani, F., Laudi, M., Pagliano, G., and Cerati, C. (1978): *Urology*, 45:595–604.

Role of Medroxyprogesterone in Endocrine-
Related Tumors, Volume II, edited by L.
Campio, G. Robustelli Della Cuna, and R. W.
Taylor. Raven Press, New York © 1983.

Medroxyprogesterone Acetate Treatment in Urological Tumors

J. Frick, R. Köhle, and H. Joos

Urological Department, General Hospital Salzburg, Salzburg, Austria

Medroxyprogesterone acetate (MPA) is a potent progestational agent which inhibits the pituitary-gonadal axis (10,15) and this compound has been used for some time in the treatment of endometrial adenocarcinoma, prostatic carcinoma, and advanced breast cancer with some success (4,6,16). In our department MPA has been employed for the treatment of two types of advanced tumors of the urogenital tract: (a) renal cell carcinoma and (b) carcinoma of the prostate.

It is assumed that about 50% of the renal cell carcinoma may present estrogen and in some percentage testosterone receptors. However it is unclear what is the pattern of receptors in their metastases. The rationale for the hormone therapy in renal cell carcinoma might be based on the assumption that the antihormone inhibits the tumor growth or at best causes a regression of the tumor metastases by blocking the receptor sites of the hormone with which it is competing (13). Though not fully proven it is almost certain that estrogen receptor synthesis is stimulated by E_2 itself and is depressed or inhibited by E_3, progestins, and antiestrogenic agents (11,13).

MATERIAL AND METHODS

Renal Cell Carcinoma

Our study for MPA treatment of certain types of renal cell carcinoma should be seen as a pure pilot study. There was neither randomization nor were receptor assays planned and performed. As this additional hormonal treatment of advanced renal cell carcinoma was first started 3 years ago, it would be too early to say anything about a significant improvement of survival rates and living quality or reduction of undue side effects.

Between January 1, 1978 and May 1981, 26 out of 53 patients with renal cell carcinoma stage III and IV (either tumor growth into the renal vein or distant metastases) who were referred to our department entered this pilot trial. The patient characteristics were as follows: stage I-II (30 patients: mean age 60.53, 18 males, 12 females); stage III-IV (53 patients: mean age 57.76, males 40, females 13).

Three weeks after transperitoneal tumor nephrectomy, removal of the adrenal gland and the retroperitoneal fat, and following clinical and pathological classification of the stage of the disease, we initiated in these 26 patients the MPA treatment in the following regimen: (a) loading dose: 1000 mg i.m. 3 times/week for 2–3 weeks; (b) maintenance dose: 1000 mg MPA i.m. every 3 weeks.

After initiation of the proposed hormonal therapy clinical examinations were conducted every 3 months. Before initiation of therapy and during each control visit the following examinations were carried out:

1. Clinical examination.

2. Urine analysis, blood samples for SMA 12 (total protein, albumin, total calcium, inorganic phosphorus, urea nitrogen, total bilirubin, alkaline phosphatase, LDH, SGPT, SGOT, and true glucose), complete blood counts, and sedimentation rate. In a few selected subjects plasma hormone determinations of LH, FSH, prolactin, testosterone, 17-β-estradiol, progesterone, and MPA. The plasma hormone analyses were done by radioimmunoassays (3,5,9,12).

3. Chest X-ray and sonography of the retroperitoneal space on the operated side including the upper abdomen above all the liver.

Before initiation of therapy and afterwards, two times per year, the following additional examinations were performed:

1. Intravenous pyelogram
2. Skeletal survey
3. Computed tomography

Table 1 summarizes the MPA-treated patients who are still under control and those who have already died. All subjects in stage III of the disease are still alive and are doing very well. The clinical and most of the laboratory parameters remained within the normal limits; the prior mentioned X-ray examinations showed no deterioration.

From the patients in stage IV, however, 33% have already died. These were cases with a far-advanced tumor stage from the very beginning. Even in these patients the MPA treatment presented some general beneficial effects such as temporary weight increase and improved sense of well being. Out of the remaining 12 patients, we found in 50% a real improvement of the disease with stabilization,

TABLE 1. *Outcome of patients with renal cell carcinoma treated with MPA after nephrectomy*

Stage	In Control		Died	
III	3M	5F	0	0
IV	11M	1F	4M	2F

regression or disappearance of the metastases, and normalization of the clinical and laboratory parameters. All these patients feel healthy and are in good general condition; in all cases an increase in body weight up to 5 kg of the pretreatment levels took place and has been maintained.

Table 2 demonstrates a typical example for the behavior of the basal hormone plasma levels seen in these MPA-treated patients: for most parameters, the values of the measured circulating hormones are decreased or remain on the lower limit of the normal range.

A regression of lung metastases in a female patient (S. W. 71 yrs), which might be due to MPA treatment, is shown in Fig. 1. We made a similar observation in 3 other cases, in 2 with lung metastases and in 1 with bone manifestation.

In summary, one should emphasize the pilot-study-like character of the trial without any randomization and the lack of receptor assays, and further one should not draw any positive or negative conclusions from these observations.

Carcinoma of the Prostate

The treatment of a disease can best be planned if we are aware of its natural history. As far as the prostate is concerned, many of the features of the disease are a consequence of its anatomical location and others are a consequence of the variation in the biological behavior of the tumor.

There are two main groups of prostatic glands, the inner and the outer. Benign prostatic hypertrophy (BPH) arises in the inner periurethral glandular tissues. Hyperplastic tissue is composed at least of epithelial and stromal tissue, but at the present time it is unclear whether both of these elements are under the same hormonal control. However, based on studies in patients following castration or treatment with progestins, it is known that at least the epithelial cells are under the control of hormones.

Attramadal and co-workers have demonstrated that the metabolic conversion of H^3-testosterone in slices of prostatic tissue showing hyperplasia is very similar to that seen in the different parts of the normal prostate. On the other hand it can be shown that the transformation of testosterone to dihydrotesterone is significantly

TABLE 2. *Behavior of plasma hormone levels
in a patient with renal cell carcinoma
treated with MPA (St. J. 69-year-old male)*

	Basal values	>6 months after MPA
LH	4.20 ng/ml	0.60 ng/ml
FSH	3.80 ng/ml	2.10 ng/ml
T	2.10 ng/ml	0.20 ng/ml
E_2	42.00 pg/ml	12.00 pg/ml
Prol.	20.00 ng/ml	18.70 ng/ml
Prog.	0.12 ng/ml	0.09 ng/ml

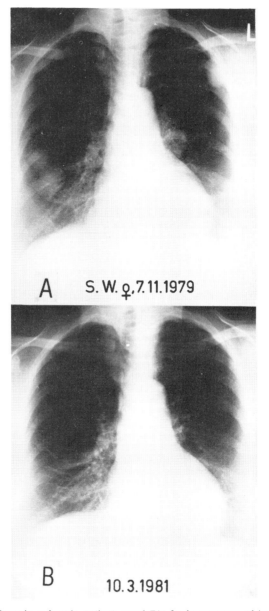

FIG. 1. Chest X-ray in a female patient, aged 71: **A:** Appearance of lung metastases 21 months after tumor nephrectomy on the left side. We initiated the proposed MPA treatment. **B:** Chest X-ray 16 months later: the lung metastases disappeared completely.

slower in prostatic cancer than in BPH or normal prostatic tissue (1,7). This might be due to the fact that a more anaplastic tissue loses some specific properties of a well-differentiated carcinoma cell, in this case the conversion of hormones to more active metabolites.

Attramadal and his group also found that the adhesion to human androgen receptors or transport proteins can be prevented by progestins (1). The therapeutic modalities of the carcinoma of the prostate have to be seen in the light of the preceding remarks. Before initiation of any treatment one should know which tumor is going to be treated and how. Under the microscope and to the naked eye all types of prostatic carcinoma are very similar. However, biologically two types can be distinguished: active or clinical cancer and latent or unsuspected cancer. In the Western world, active tumors are found in about 16 per 100,000 cases. Close to 30% of all men over 50 years of age have a latent or retarded carcinoma of the prostate. These lesions are indistinguishable histologically from active clinical tumors; however, they do not grow or kill the patients.

The results of therapy of prostatic cancer must be appraised against the biological and pathological background. But how do we know how any given tumor is going to behave? The differentiation between a low or high degree of biological malignancy is a problem that needs to be solved. At the moment one can say only that patients with well-differentiated tumors will have a better prognosis than a group with anaplastic tumors.

If a carcinoma of the prostate responds to endocrine therapy, the tumor is referred to as hormone sensitive. However, this term can only be applied to those parts of the tumor which respond, and not to the whole tumor. Even in the same tumor one can find degenerative changes and undamaged cells very close together. Hormone sensitivity may not be a property of the whole tumor but may vary from part to part of the same tumor.

The percentage of patients with tumors entirely confined to the gland is very small. To perform radical surgery in these cases might be a logical treatment (14). The greater number of patients, however, are suitable for different forms of general treatment: surgery, internal or external radiation, or hormonal therapy depending upon the stage and grade of the disease (8,18). To stage the tumor before initiation of treatment is very important, and for this a number of examinations have to be carried out. Namely: rectal palpation, i.v. urogram, urethrocystogram, chest roentgenogram, bone X-ray, bone scan, lymphangiography, sonography of the lymph nodes, CAT, phosphatase plasma levels, hormone plasma levels. This list might be incomplete and the measurements of sex steroid binding globulin and receptor studies should probably be added.

The classification is finally done according to Flocks:

Stage A: lesion completely limited to prostate;
Stage B: lesion involving most of the prostate;
Stage C: lesion locally extended beyond prostate to regions of the base of the bladder and seminal vesicles;
Stage D: lesions clinically disseminated to lymph nodes and to bones.

A fragmentary list of the therapeutic modalities for the different stages of prostatic cancer can be summarized as follows:

Stage A: observation, TUR, radical prostatectomy with lymphadenectomy, open perineal cryosurgery with lymphadenectomy;

Stage B: radical prostatectomy with lymphadenectomy, open perineal cryosurgery with lymphadenectomy, application of A^{198} or J^{125} with lymphadenectomy, radiation;

Stage C: application of A^{198} or J^{125} with lymphadenectomy, radical prostatectomy or open perineal cryosurgery with lymphadenectomy, intraurethral or external radiation, endocrine therapy;

Stage D: endocrine therapy, palliative TUR, radiation (primary lesion and metastases).

The endocrine therapy for carcinoma of the prostate has to be initiated with a view of suppression of androgen production, of changing the hormonal environment, and of influencing the metabolism of the prostatic cells by progestin administration (see, for example, ref. 2).

Hormonal treatment might be undertaken in different ways: orchidectomy, low-dose hormonal therapy, high-dose hormonal treatment, long-term hormone therapy, interval therapy, adrenalectomy and hypophysectomy.

The life-long treatment, the often unpredictable course of the disease, the onset of a second disease, or the evidence of side effects during hormonal treatment create a number of problems that have to be considered. A successful endocrine treatment is only possible, provided the treated patient cooperates and fulfills the intended protocol.

Three years ago we initiated a pilot study with MPA in 17 patients with an average age of 72.6 years who were suffering from prostatic cancer, stage C and D. This was just less than 10% of the whole prostatic cancer material during that time period. The therapeutic regimen was the same as for the renal cell carcinoma: loading dose of 500–1000 mg MPA 3 times/week for 2–3 weeks, maintenance dose of 1000 mg MPA every third week. The parameters measured before initiation and during treatment at regular intervals were the same as previously shown for MPA treatment in patients with renal cell carcinoma.

Table 3 shows a fragmentary synopsis of the findings in regard to chest X-ray, acid phosphatases, and local extension during the treatment. In 5 out of 17 patients a deterioration in one or two of these parameters took place, but in summary one has to mention that all these patients are still alive and even those who had a progression of the disease showed subjective well being.

TABLE 3.   *Prostatic cancer, stage C and D (MPA treatment; N = 17)*

	Chest X-ray	Phosphatases	Local findings
Normal, stationary, or improved	16	11	12
Deteriorated	1	6	5

It would be too early and too misleading to draw any conclusions from this pilot study, although the response of some prostatic cancer patients to progestin treatment is sometimes dramatic. Clinically, primary and secondary tumors may become progressively smaller. Patients also react to progestin therapy very well: they show fewer side effects compared with those associated with estrogen preparations used previously, such as development of gynecomastia, cardiovascular problems, and liver toxicity.

It has already been pointed out several times that the treatment of prostatic carcinoma is a subject of controversy. This fact might be based at least on three features (17): (a) the disease occurs in an age group wherein the risks of death from a variety of causes other than prostatic cancer are high and increasing. (b) The definition of the natural history of the cancer both in terms of rate of progression and pattern of progression is incomplete. (c) The therapeutic modalities vary: surgical, radiation, or endocrine, either individually or in various combinations.

REFERENCES

1. Attramadal, A., Weddington, S. C., Maess, O., Djoseland, O., and Hausson, V. (1976): *Progress in Clinical and Biological Research.* Alan R. Liss, New York.
3. Bardin, C. W. (1981): *Abstracts, Progesterone and Progestins.* International Symposium, Paris, May 7–9.
3. Bartke, A., Steele, R. E., Musto, N., and Caldwell, B. V. (1973): *Endocrinology,* 92:1223–1228.
4. Boute, J., Decoster, J. M., Ide, P., and Billiet, G. (1978): *Gynecol. Oncol.,* 6:70–79.
5. Crosignani, P. G., Nakamura, R. M., Hovland, D. N., and Mishell, D. R., Jr. (1970): *J. Clin. Endocrinol. Metab.,* 30:153–160.
6. De Lena, M., Brambilla, C., Valagussa, P., and Bonadonna, G. (1979): *Cancer Chemother. Pharmacol.,* 2:175–182.
7. Fang, S., and Liao, S. (1971): *J. Biol. Chem.,* 246:16–24.
8. Flocks, R. H. (1969): *JAMA,* 210:328–337.
9. Frick, J., Bartsch, G., and Jakse, G. (1977): *Urol. Res.,* 5:55–59.
10. Frick, J., Bartsch, G., and Weiske, W. H. (1977): *Contraception,* 6:649–668.
11. Gurpide, E. (1976): *Cancer,* 38:503–509.
12. Hotchkiss, J., Atkinson, L. E., and Knobil, E. (1971): *Endocrinology,* 89:177–183.
13. Ilsueh, A. J. W., Peck, I. J., Jr., and Clark, J. H. (1975): *Nature,* 254:337–348.
14. Jewett, H. J. (1975): *Urol. Clin. North Am.,* 2:105–112.
15. Meyer, W. J., Walker, P. A., Wiedeking, C., Money, J., and Kowarski, A. A. (1977): *Fertil. Steril.,* 28:1072–1081.
16. Rafla, S., and Johonson, R. (1974): *Curr. Ther. Res.,* 16:261–269.
17. Whitmore, W. F. (1973): *Cancer,* 32:1104–1114.
18. Whitmore, W. F., Hilaris, B., and Grabstald, H. (1972): *J. Urol.,* 108:918–929.

Role of Medroxyprogesterone in Endocrine-Related Tumors, Volume II, edited by L. Campio, G. Robustelli Della Cuna, and R. W. Taylor. Raven Press, New York © 1983.

Steroid Receptors and Human Renal Cell Carcinoma

Franco Di Silverio and *Giuseppe Concolino

*Department of Urology, Division of Urological Pathology, and *Fifth Institute of General Clinical Medicine and Therapy, University of Rome, 00161 Rome, Italy*

In the last decade tumors arising from human endometrial, mammary, and prostatic tissues as well as leukemia, renal cell carcinoma (RCC), laringopharingeal cancer, melanoma, and colorectal cancer have been considered hormone-related and in some instances hormone-responsive (6,10,23). The concept of hormone-dependent tumors was derived from evidence of experimental tumor models induced by prolonged administration of hormones (22,24,25,30,33), evidence of lack of induction of tumor in experimental animals by the addition of a hormonal antagonist, evidence of regression or stabilization of the tumor in man following endocrine manipulation, and evidence of hormone receptors in carcinoma as a biochemical marker for hormone dependence both in animals and man (8,9,12,15).

It is well known that steroid hormones act on target tissues such as endometrial, mammary, and prostatic tissues (13,14,17). Various hormones including mineralo- and glucocorticoids as well as calcitonin and vitamin D act on renal tissue (16). Sex steroids also act upon the renal cell, e.g., estrogens and androgens induce morphological and biochemical changes of opposite type (34). The existence of a sex influence on renal tumorigenesis is supported by the finding that male dogs are more frequently affected by RCC than the female. Furthermore, in Syrian hamsters, RCC can be induced with prolonged estrogen administration in the male, or in the female ovariectomized animal (23,25).

TABLE 1. *Effect of TAM[a] on PR in normal human kidney and in human renal cell carcinoma*

	PR (fmol/mg prot.)	
	No treatment	TAM
Normal kidney tissue	2.96	66.13
RCC	4.09 ± 2.81	16.43 ± 4.05

[a]Patients treated with tamoxifen (20 mg/p.d. for 7 days) before surgery.

The best experimental model of RCC is that induced by long-term treatment with natural or synthetic estrogens in the male Syrian hamster and the castrated female: RCC are often bilateral with multiple tumors arising from the tubular epithelium. These RCC have a high degree of malignancy with metastasis in the lymph nodes and lungs. Furthermore, the histological pattern of these tumors resembles adenocarcinoma in humans with high content of lipophilic material in the neoplastic cells (5,6,26–28).

As far as hormone sensitivity is concerned, full growth of these tumors requires the presence of estrogens, while progesterone plus cortisone produces marked tumor inhibition.

The tumor can be transplanted into other hamsters pretreated with estrogens or androgens. Therefore there is plenty of evidence that renal cancer, in some laboratory animals, is hormone dependent. In RCC of Syrian hamster Li et al. reported the presence of estradiol (ER), progesterone (PR), and androgen receptors (AR): PR concentration, in response to estrogen treatment, increases in renal tissue 17- to 27-fold untreated control levels, and in the estrogen-induced tumor becomes 520 times higher than that in control animals. Progesterone treatment reduces specific ER in the tumor (29,30,31).

In man, a relationship has been demonstrated between hormones and tumor growth rate in many neoplasias. The hypothesis of hormone dependence of RCC in man is based on sex differences (male to female ratio being 3.8:1); racial differences (RCC is frequently found in whites but seldom in blacks); differences in hormonal status could explain the more frequent regression of RCC in women than in men and the regression of RCC found in the presence of adrenal tumor (1,2,4,32). On the basis of these considerations, steroid receptors have been studied in normal human renal tissue and human RCC in order to explain the action of steroid hormones in the urological tract and hormone sensitivity of urological neoplasias.

In the last few years cytoplasmic and nuclear ER, PR, and AR are being identified in the human RCC: our investigations have been focused in particular on the meaning of nuclear AR as a marker of hormone responsiveness to pharmacological doses of medroxyprogesterone acetate (MPA). Furthermore, we have preliminary data show-

TABLE 2. *Distribution of steroid receptors (ER, PR, and AR) in pT_2 and pT_3 patients*

	pT_2		pT_3	
Receptors	N	(%)	N	(%)
ER+	20	58.9	9	56.2
ER−	14	41.1	7	43.8
PR+	20	58.9	10	62.5
PR−	14	41.1	6	37.5
AR+	9	64.3	7	70.0
AR−	5	35.7	3	10.0

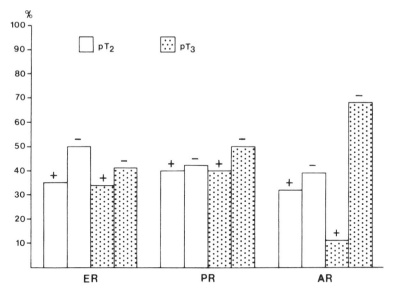

FIG. 1. Steroid receptors and death rate in pT_2 and pT_3 patients.

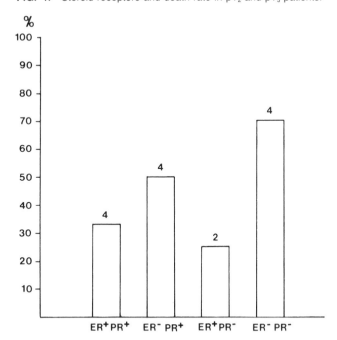

FIG. 2. Combined steroid receptors (ER and PR) and death rate in pT_2 patients.

ing an increase in PR concentration in RCC of patients treated with tamoxifen (TAM) 7 days before nephrectomy, thus providing support for the concept that the action of estradiol on RCC is mediated through the receptor mechanism (Table 1).

If all these observations led us to consider the human RCC as a hormone-dependent tumor, what clinical results have been obtained in the endocrine treatment of the carcinoma? Are the receptors markers of hormone dependence or just favorable prognostic parameters?

There are contradictory reports in the literature regarding the use both of MPA and androgen therapy (3,4,6,7,10,11,35,38,39). Antiestrogens alone do not seem to be of benefit to patients with RCC (18). Furthermore, it is worthwhile pointing out that RCC shows a low response rate to chemotherapy both with single or with combined agents. Some interesting response rates were claimed using MPA associated with chemoimmunotherapy (19–21,36,37,40).

In order to throw further light on these aspects we carried out investigations on 50 patients (mean age 61.4 years; M/F ratio 2.3:1) submitted to radical nephrectomy and treated with MPA at pharmacological doses. According to TNM classification the histological stage was pT_2 in 34 patients and pT_3 in 16. Lymph node (N_1) involvement was found in 35% of patients in both groups. Since no distant metastatic

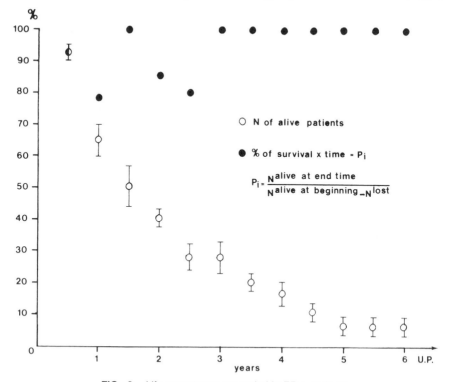

FIG. 3. Life expectancy per period in ER+ patients.

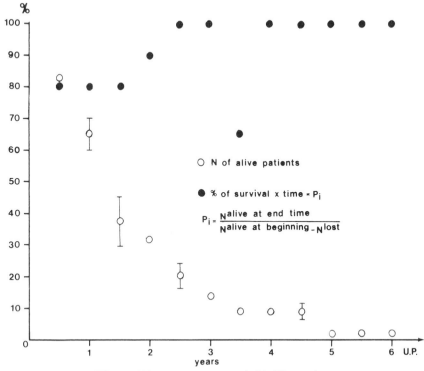

FIG. 4.   Life expectancy per period in ER − patients.

lesions (M_0) were demonstrated, death rate, survival, and life expectancy were studied with regard to receptor data.

The distribution of steroid receptors in two groups of patients shows a slight increase in the percentage of receptor-positive cancers both in the pT_2 and pT_3 groups (Table 2).

CORRELATION BETWEEN HISTOLOGICAL STAGE, RECEPTORS, AND DEATH RATE

Preliminary analysis of the data emerging from the present study (Fig. 1) reveals that the death rate is higher in the patients with receptor-negative cancers regardless of the steroid receptors and histological stage considered. Within 36 months, in fact, 50% of the ER − patients died, while 35% of the ER + patients died, i.e., the death rate is lower in patients with receptor-positive cancers. This observation is more clearly demonstrated when the combined ER are considered. In fact, as shown in Fig. 2 the highest death rate (66%) occurs in the group of pT_2 patients with ER − PR − RCC, while in the ER + PR −, ER − PR +, ER + PR + groups, the mean death rate is 37%. This correlation could not be demonstrated in the pT_3 group on account of the limited number of patients.

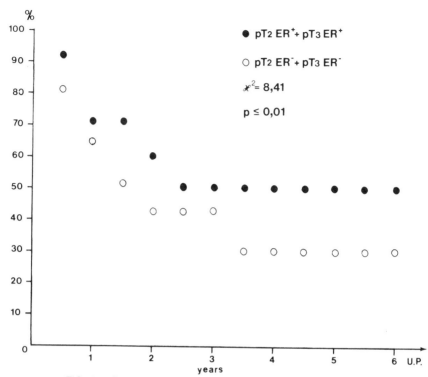

FIG. 5. Overall life expectancy of the group with and without ER.

TABLE 3.   *Deaths per period/patients present at the*
beginning of the follow-up period
(ratio in the ER+ and ER−group)

Months	ER +	ER −	Confidence level (%)
12	7/29	7/21	$\simeq 40$
18	7/29	9/21	$\simeq 25$
24	9/29	10/21	$\simeq 30$
30	10/29	10/21	$\simeq 35$

CORRELATION BETWEEN HISTOLOGICAL STAGE (pT_2–pT_3), RECEPTORS AND PROBABILITY OF SURVIVAL

In these 50 patients, observed between 1975 and 1980, with a follow-up period ranging between 6 months and 6 years, death occurred in 20 (40%). It is not possible, on the basis of the data obtained, to prepare an actuarial curve of survival, inasmuch as the latter, to be sufficiently reliable should refer to a larger number of observations, a homogeneous follow-up period, and a larger number of patients. Nevertheless, calculations were made of the life expectancy per period and overall life expectancy. It should be pointed out, however, that even if standard errors were assumed in

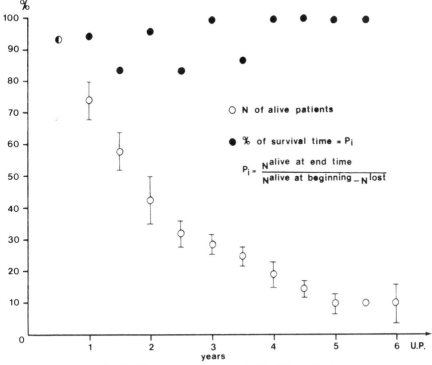

FIG. 6. Life expectancy per period in PR+ patients.

these calculations, the results cannot be considered reliable on account of the limited number of patients studied.

A comparison was made between ER+ patients, PR+ patients, and the respective negative groups. ER+ and probability of the survival are reported in Fig. 3, which also shows the number of patients still alive in each period under consideration, as well as the probability of survival for that period. The latter is calculated by dividing the number of patients alive at the end of the period by the number alive at the beginning minus the number of cases no longer in the follow-up study. Death occurs within the first 30 months and the life expectancy in that period is about 85%. As far as ER− patients are concerned, most deaths occur within the first 24 months with a life expectancy ranging between 80 and 90%, whereas at 42 months life expectancy drops to 65% (Fig. 4).

The prognostic value of ER is confirmed by the results reported in Fig. 5, which shows the overall life expectancy of the groups with and without ER. It can be seen that, as far as the life expectancy beyond the third year is concerned, the presence of ER shows a favorable prognostic significance.

Considering the wide margin of error of our statistics, we also calculated the number of deaths per period out of the number of patients present at the beginning of the follow-up period and the confidence level. The latter expresses the casual

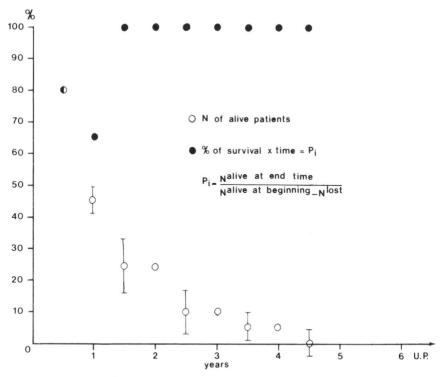

FIG. 7. Life expectancy per period in PR − patients.

life expectancy, i.e., the probability that two samples belong to completely different populations and not to the same populations. A difference exists between the two groups both in the absolute number of deaths per period and the overall number (Table 3). However the confidence level suggests caution in the interpretation of these data.

Data from the group of patients with PR + are given in Fig. 6. Deaths are fairly uniformly distributed in the first 36 months, with a life expectancy per period of about 90%. From data obtained in the PR − patients (Fig. 7), it has been demonstrated that all deaths occur within the first 12 months, with a mean life expectancy per period of about 70%. When the overall life expectancy is taken into consideration (Fig. 8), the prognostic importance of the progesterone receptors with the first 2 years appears evident, whereas in the next phase values coincide. Also in this instance calculations were made of the number of deaths per period out of the number of patients at the beginning of the follow-up observation, extrapolating the statistical significance with relative confidence level (Table 4). Statistical differences were observed particularly at 12 and 18 months. The very low confidence level provides an excellent safety margin on the statistical reliability of data from the first two periods under examination.

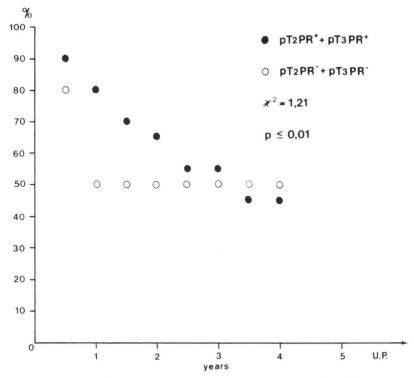

FIG. 8. Overall life expectancy of the group with and without PR.

TABLE 4. *Deaths per period/patients present at the beginning of the follow-up period (ratio in the PR+ and PR− groups)*

Months	PR +	PR −	Confidence level (%)
12	5/30	9/20	$\approx$ 3.5
18	8/30	9/20	$\approx$ 17.0
24	9/30	9/20	$\approx$ 30.0
30	11/30	9/20	$\approx$ 50.0

CONCLUSIONS

In conclusion, the presence of steroid receptors in human RCC, the favorable effect of hormone treatment in receptor-positive cancer, and the prognostic value of steroid receptors led us to consider that human RCC is also a hormone-dependent tumor. Furthermore, the favorable prognostic significance of the progesterone receptor may be reasonably substantiated, particularly as far as life expectancy at 12 and 18 months is concerned.

With regard to the estrogen receptor, on the other hand, the available data should be evaluated with caution even if this appears to have a certain prognostic significance on a longer probability of survival.

Studies on a larger number of cases with a longer and more homogeneous follow-up period may provide data in support of findings emerging from the present investigation.

ACKNOWLEDGMENTS

This work was supported in part by a grant of C.N.R. (Italy) Special Project "Control of neoplastic growth." The collaboration of Drs. R. Tenaglia, E. Pannunzio, A. Fagioli, G. D'Eramo, and E. Cruciani in the elaboration of the data and preparation of this report is gratefully acknowledged.

REFERENCES

1. Bartley, O., and Hulquist, G. T. (1950): *Acta Pathol. Microbiol. Scand.*, 27:448.
2. Bennington, J. L. (1973): *Cancer*, 32:1017.
3. Bloom, H. J. G. (1971): *Br. J. Cancer*, 25:205.
4. Bloom, H. J. G. (1973): *Cancer*, 32:1066–1071.
5. Bloom, H. J. G., Baker, W. H., Dukes, C. E., and Mitchley, B. C. V. (1963): *Br. J. Cancer*, 17:646.
6. Bloom, H. J. G., Duker, C. E., and Mitchley, B. C. V. (1963): *Br. J. Cancer*, 17:611–645.
7. Bloom, H. J. G., and Wallace, D. M. (1964): *Br. Med. J.*, 2:476.
8. Bojar, H., Wittliff, J. L., Balser, K., Dreyfurst, R., Boenïnghans, F., and Staib, W. (1975): *Acta Endocrinol. (Kbh), Suppl.*, 193:51.
9. Bojar, H., Dreyfurst, R., Baller, K., Staib, W., and Wittliff, J. L. (1976): *J. Clin. Chem. Clin. Biochem.*, 14:521–526.
10. Bracci, U., and Di Silverio, F. (1976): *Atti XLIX Congresso S.I.U.*, Vol. I, p. 167. Ferrara, Italy.
11. Bracci, U., Gagliardi, V., and Di Silverio, F. (1973): In: *Proc. XVI Congress of Int. Soc. Urol.*, Vol. 2, p. 569. Doin, Paris.
12. Concolino, G., Marocchi, A., Martelli, M. L., Gagliardi, V., and Di Silverio, F. (1975): *J. Steroid Biochem.*, 6:XV.
13. Concolino, G., Di Silverio, F., Marocchi, A., Tenaglia, R., and Bracci, U. (1979): In: *Proceedings X Congress of the European Federation of the International College of Surgeons*, edited by Minerva Medica, pp. 383–387. Turin, Italy.
14. Concolino, G., Marocchi, A., Conti, C., Liberti, M., Tenaglia, R., and Di Silverio, F. (1980): In: *Hormones and Cancer*, edited by S. Iacobelli et al. Raven Press, New York.
15. Concolino, G., Marocchi, A., Di Silverio, F., and Conti, C. (1976): *J. Steroid Biochem.*, 7:923.
16. Di Silverio, F., Gallucci, M., Cruciani, E., Ferrone, G., and Mussini, M. (1981): *Simposio nazionale su: Calcitonina acquisizioni e prospettive*. Venice, Italy *(Abstr.)*.
17. Fanestil, D. D., Vaughn, D. A., and Ludens, J. H. (1974): *J. Steroid Biochem.*, 5:338.
18. Glick, J. et al. (1979): In:s36*Proc. Am. Assoc. Cancer Res. and Am. Soc. Clin. Oncol.*, 20:311.
19. Hahn, D. M. et al. (1977): *Cancer Treat. Rep.*, 61:1585.
20. Hahn, R. G. et al. (1978): *Cancer Treat. Rep.*, 62:1093.
21. Hire, E. A. et al. (1979): *Cancer Clin. Trials*, 2:293.
22. Horning, E. (1956): *Br. J. Cancer*, 10:678–687.
23. Horning, E. S. (1956): *Z. Krebsforschung*, 61:1–4.
24. Kirkman, H. (1959): *Natl. Cancer Inst. Monogr.*, 1:1–139.
25. Letourneau, R. J., Li, J. J., Rosen, S., and Villee, C. A. (1975): *Cancer Res.*, 35:6–10.
26. Li, J. J., and Li, S. A. (1975): *Am. Assoc. Cancer Res. Int. Annual Meeting*, San Diego, California *(Abstr.)*.
27. Li, J. J., and Li, S. A. (1977): In: *Research on Steroids*, Vol. VII, edited by Vermeulen et al. North Holland, Amsterdam.
28. Li, S. A., and Li, J. J. (1975): *The Endocrine Society, (abstr.)*, New York.

29. Li, J. J., Li, S. A., Merry, B. J., and Villee, C. A. (1974): *J. Steroid Biochem.*, 5:340.
30. Li, J. J., Tolley, D. J., Li, S. A., and Villee, C. A. (1974): *Endocrinology*, 95:1134–1141.
31. Li, J. J., Tolley, D. J., Li, S. A., and Villee, C. A. (1976): *Cancer Res.*, 36:1127–1132.
32. Kantor, A. L. F., Meigs, J. M., Heston, J. F., and Flannery, J. T. (1976): *J. Natl. Cancer Inst.*, 57:495.
33. Matthews, V. S., Kirkman, H., and Bacon, R. L. (1947): *Proc. Soc. Exp. Biol. Med.*, 66:195–201.
34. Matulich, D. T., Spindler, B. J., Schambelan, M., and Baxter, J. D. (1976): *J. Clin. Endocrinol. Metab.*, 43:1170–1174.
35. Paine, C. H., Wright, F. W., and Ellis, F. (1970): *Br. J. Cancer*, 24:277.
36. Pasmantier, M. W. et al. (1977): *Cancer Treat. Rep.*, 61:1731.
37. Rodriguez, L. H., and Johnson, D. E. (1978): *Urology*, 11:344.
38. Samuels, M. L., Sullivan, P., and Hawe, C. D. (1968): *Cancer*, 22:523–532.
39. Wagle, D. G., and Murphy, G. P. (1971): *Cancer*, 28:318.
40. Wong, P. P., et al. (1977): *Cancer Treat. Rep.*, 61:1727.

Subject Index

Adenocarcinoma
  cure rate, 148
  differentiation in, 141–142, 144,
    146, 152
  estradiol and, 142–143, 152
  estrogens and, 141–142, 152
  hormone dependency of,
    141–142, 152
  MPA and, 145, 147, 152–155,
    169–170
  progesterone receptor in,
    146–147, 152
  progestogens and, 144–146
  radiotherapy of, 147–151
  remission of, 147, 150–152
  surgery for, 148
  TAM and, 152–155
Adrenocorticotropic hormone
  (ACTH), MPA and, 105, 125
Adriamycin
  in breast cancer, 89–91, 135,
    137
  MPA and, 89–91
  toxicity of, 89, 137
Age factors
  in breast cancer, 73
  in endometrial carcinoma, 168,
    169
Aminoglutethimide
  in breast cancer, 62, 91–92
  MPA and, 91–92
  side effects, 91–92
  therapeutics of, 92
Androgens
  in renal cell carcinoma, 199–200
  receptors for, 199–200

Breast cancer
  advanced, 69–74, 77–82, 115–127
  age and, 73
  aminoglutethimide in, 62, 91–92
  bromocriptine in, 115–127
  cell culture of, 1–4
  chemotherapy combinations in,
    85–93, 112, 131–138
  cytotoxic agents in, 131
  estrogen in, 15, 48, 53, 64
  hormonal treatment in, 45–48,
    63–65
  metastasis in, 50, 55, 78, 79–80,
    91, 95–103, 116
  mitomycin in, 85–89
  MPA in, 1–5, 17, 35, 57–66,
    69–74, 77–82, 85–93,
    95–103, 109, 117
  multidrug regimen in, 131–138
  ovariectomy in, 49, 56, 62
  pain in, 60, 62, 99, 101–102
  patient characteristics in, 86–87
  postmenopausal, 70–74, 95–103
  progestin in, 16–17, 47, 53
  prolactin in, 53, 115, 119, 122
  radiotherapy in, 112
  receptors in, 15, 45, 46, 60–61,
    63, 73, 116–119, 127, 131
  response criteria, 110,117
  response duration in, 45
  response rate in, 45, 58, 69, 70,
    71–74, 78–82, 96–97,
    108–111
  stage IV studies of, 115, 124
  TAM in, 15–17, 47–66, 133,
    135, 137

Breast cancer *(contd.)*
　therapeutic strategy in, 60–65
Bromocriptine
　in breast cancer, 115–127
　dopamine and, 124–125
　mechanism of action, 124–125
　MPA and, 115–127
　prolactin and, 115, 124
　receptors and, 115–119
　response to, 117–118, 120–121,
　　127
　side effects, of, 119, 123
　treatment schedule, 117

Cell culture
　of CG-5 cells, 1–5
　of endometrial carcinoma, 142
　of MCF-7 cells, 1, 4–5
Cell cycle
　DNA synthesis and, 7
　menstruation and, 8–9
CG-5 cells
　hormone receptors in, 1
　MPA and, 1–5
　TAM and, 2–5
Clomiphene, in breast cancer,
　47–48
Cortisol, in breast cancer, 119, 122
Cutaneous metastases, in breast
　　cancer, 16
Cyclophosphamide, in breast
　　cancer, 132–133, 135, 137
Cyproterone acetate, in prostatic
　　cancer, 184–190
Cytoxane
　in breast cancer, 89–91
　MPA and, 89–91

Dehydroepiandrosterone sulfate, in
　　breast cancer, 116, 119
Diethylstilbestrol
　in breast cancer, 132

　in prostatic cancer, 184–190
DNA-dependent RNA polymerase,
　　TAM and, 49
DNA synthesis
　cell cycle and, 7–13
　flow cytometry and, 8
　in ovarian tumors, 177
Dopamine, bromocriptine and,
　　124–125

Endometrial carcinoma
　as adenocarcinoma, 169,
　　171–172
　adjuvant therapy of, 158,
　　166–167
　age factor in, 168–169
　cure rate of, 157, 160
　differentiation in, 160, 169,
　　171–172
　hormone dependency of,
　　141–142, 157
　hysterectomy in, 167, 172
　in vitro studies of, 142
　lymph node metastases in,
　　164–165, 169–170
　MPA in, 20–24, 25–34,
　　157–162, 169–170
　myometrial invasion in, 160,
　　163–164
　radiotherapy in, 157, 161, 166
　remission rate in, 157–161
　stage I studies, 163–172
　steroid hormone enzyme
　　induction in, 161–162
　surgical treatment of, 166, 167,
　　172
Endometrium
　adenocarcinoma of, 8, 10–12
　carcinoma of, 10–12, 20–24,
　　25–34
　cell cycle in, 7
　DNA synthesis in, 7–13
　estrogens in, 144, 157

flow cytometry in, 7–13
hyperplasia in, 10
in menstruation, 7–13
MPA and, 8–13
progesterone and, 157–158
Estradiol
in adenocarcinoma, 142–143
in breast cancer, 15
endometrium and, 49
MPA and, 2–3, 48, 52, 124, 126
in ovarian cancer, 177
receptors, 15
TAM and, 48–49, 152
Estramustine phosphate, in
prostatic cancer, 184, 189
Estrogen
adenocarcinoma and, 141–142,
152
antagonists of, 158
breast cancer and, 15, 17, 48–54
in endometrial carcinoma, 144,
157
progestin and, 105
prolactin and, 48–49
in prostatic cancer, 183
receptors, 105, 144–145, 155,
157
in renal cell carcinoma, 199–200
TAM and, 15, 152

Farlutal, versus Provera, 20, 23
Fluorouracil, in breast cancer,
132–133
Follicle-stimulating hormone (FSH)
in adenocarcinoma, 142–143
in breast cancer, 71, 116, 119,
123
MPA and, 105, 125, 145
TAM and, 152

Hypercalcemia, TAM and, 57

Hyperprolactinemia, in breast
cancer, 91
Hypophyseal gonadotrpins,
progestins and, 54
Hypophysectomy
in breast cancer, 65–66
TAM and, 65
Hysterectomy, in endometrial
carcinoma, 167, 172

Luteinizing hormone (LH)
in adenocarcinoma, 142–143
in breast cancer, 71, 116, 119
123
MPA and, 105, 125, 184
TAM and, 152

Medroxyprogesterone acetate
(MPA)
in adenocarcinoma, 145, 147,
153–155, 169–170
administration schedules, 35–36
antiestrogenic effects, 1
body weight and, 99–100
bone marrow toxicity and, 54,
90–91, 180
breast cancer and, 1–5, 17, 35,
57–66, 69–74, 77–82,
85–93, 95–103, 109, 117
bromocriptine and, 115–127
cell proliferation and, 1–5
in CG-5 cells, 1–5
chemotherapy combination, 59,
80, 82, 85–93, 112,
178–180
dose levels, 25–34, 35–36, 48,
69–74, 77–82, 85, 95–100,
117, 133
in endometrial carcinoma,
20–24, 25–34, 52,
157–162, 169–170
endometrium and, 8–13

MPA *(contd.)*
  estradiol and, 2–3, 5, 48, 52,
    124, 126
  estrogens and, 17, 48–54
  FSH and, 105, 125, 145
  hyperplasia and, 10–12
  intramuscular, 25–28, 31–34,
    95–96, 106
  LH and, 105, 125, 184
  mechanism of action, 51–55, 77,
    105–106
  menopause and, 95–103, 111
  metabolism of, 27
  metastases and, 78, 91, 95–103
  mitomycin and, 85–89
  oral administration of, 19–24,
    28–34, 36, 95–103, 106
  in ovarian cancer, 177–180
  pain and, 39, 41–42, 60, 99,
    101–102
  pharmacodynamics of, 97–98
  pharmacokinetics of, 19–24,
    25–34, 103
  pharmacology of, 106–109
  phase II studies, 85–93
  pituitary and, 124
  plasma levels of, 20–24, 25–34,
    35–43, 103
  in postmenopausal patients, 5,
    70–74, 95–103
  progestogen and, 153–154
  prolactin and, 52
  in prostatic cancer, 183–190,
    196
  radioimmunoassay of, 21–22, 27
  in renal cell carcinoma, 191–193
  response rate to, 39–42, 58–59,
    69, 71–74, 78–82, 89–90,
    96–103, 108–111, 151
  side effects of, 59–60, 65, 73,
    80, 87, 89–91, 97, 103, 111
  TAM and, 2–5, 57–66, 133–138
  time/concentration curves for,
    37–38

  toxicity of, 80–81
  in urine, 23
  for urological tumors, 191–197
Menopause
  breast cancer and, 95–103, 111,
    116, 132
  cancer remission and, 98
Menstrual cycle
  cell cycle and, 8–9
  endometrium in, 7–9
Menstruation, DNA flow cytometry
  in 7–13
Metastases
  in breast cancer, 16, 50, 55, 78,
    79–80, 91, 95–103, 116
  cutaneous, 16
  in endometrial carcinoma,
    163–165
  in lymph nodes, 164–166,
    169–170
  MPA and, 78, 91, 95–103
  risk factors in, 53, 97–98
  site of, 79–80
  TAM and, 16, 50, 55–56
Mitomycin
  in breast cancer, 85–89
  MPA and, 85–89
  response rate, 88–89
  toxicity of, 87–88

Nafoxidine, in breast cancer, 47–
  48

Ovarian cancer
  chemotherapy in, 178–180
  epithelium in, 177–180
  estradiol in, 177
  hormonal receptors in, 177
  MPA in, 178–180
  progesterone and, 177
  remission rate, 179–180
  treatment side effects in, 180

Ovariectomy
in breast cancer, 49, 56, 62
in endometrial carcinoma, 158
TAM and, 56

Pain
MPA and, 39, 41–42, 99,
101–102
MPA plasma levels and, 39,
41–42
Progesterone
in endometrial carcinoma, 158
endometrium and, 157–158
estrogens and, 124
MPA and, 105
in ovarian cancer, 177
receptors, 1, 5, 15–16, 105,
146–147, 152, 177, 200,
204–207
in renal cell carcinoma, 200
Progestogens
in adenocarcinoma, 144, 155
administration route and, 150
in endometrial carcinoma,
158–162
estrogen receptors and, 145
MPA and, 153–155
response to, 149, 151
side effects of, 151
Prolactin
in breast cancer, 53, 115, 119,
122
bromocriptine and, 115, 124
estrogen and, 48–49
MPA and, 52
progestins and, 53
receptors, 115, 127
Prostaglandin-synthetase, TAM
and, 50
Prostatic carcinoma
cardiovascular toxicity in,
186–189
chemotherapy in, 184–190

classification of, 195–196
hormonal role in, 46, 193–194
incidence of, 195
metastasis in, 185
MPA in, 183–190, 196
progestin in, 53, 193, 195, 197
response rate, 189
treatment procedures, 183–190,
196
treatment side effects, 186–188
Prostatic hypertrophy, testosterone
in, 193–194

Radiotherapy
in adenocarcinoma, 147–151,
160
in breast cancer, 112
in endometrial carcinoma, 157,
161, 166
Receptors
in adenocarcinoma, 146–147,
152–153, 155
to androgen, 199–200
in breast cancer, 15, 45–46,
60–61, 115–119, 127, 131
in endometrial carcinoma,
142–144, 146–147
to estradiol, 15–16, 152–153,
116–117, 124, 126,
152–153, 177
to estrogen, 105, 142, 144–145,
155, 157, 191, 199, 208
MPA and, 105–106, 127
in ovarian cancer, 177
progesterone, 1, 5, 15–16, 105,
116, 146–147, 152,
200–201, 204–207
to progestin, 49
to prolactin, 115, 127
in renal cell carcinoma, 191,
199–208
to testosterone, 191

translocation of, 49
treatment response and,
117–118, 121, 127
Renal cell carcinoma
age and, 191
androgen receptors in, 199–200
death rate in, 202–207
estrogens and, 199, 200
estrogen receptors in, 191,
200–201, 208
histology, and, 203–207
MPA in, 191–193
nephrectomy in, 202
plasma hormones in, 193
progesterone receptors in,
200–201, 204–207
racial differences in, 200
response rate, 192–193,
202–207
steroid receptors in, 199–208
TAM in, 199, 202
testosterone receptors in,
191–201

Serum acid phosphate, in prostatic
cancer, 185
Sex hormone binding, in breast
cancer, 71

Tamoxifen (TAM)
in adenocarcinoma, 152–155
antiestrogenic effects, 48–51
in breast cancer, 15–17,
47–66, 133, 135, 137
chemotherapy combination, 56,
59, 133–134

cost factors in, 66
dose levels, 55–57
estradiol and, 49, 152
estradiol binding and, 48
estrogen target cells and,
15–16, 65
half-life of, 55
mechanism of action of, 48–55,
133
menopausal state and, 55, 133
metastases and, 16, 50, 55–56
MPA and, 2–5, 57–66,
133–138
plasma levels of, 55–57
progestin and, 16–17, 48, 64
properties of, 48–55
prostaglandin and, 5051
in renal cell carcinoma, 199, 202
response rate to, 55, 57, 59, 152
side effects, 48, 56, 65
therapeutic response to, 55
Testosterone
in prostatic cancer, 184
in prostatic hypertrophy,
193–194
in urological tumors, 191

Urological tumors, testosterone in,
191

Vincristine
in breast cancer, 89–91, 133
MPA and, 89–91